Charles Kingsley

Health and education

Charles Kingsley

Health and education

ISBN/EAN: 9783337215125

Printed in Europe, USA, Canada, Australia, Japan

Cover: Foto ©Andreas Hilbeck / pixelio.de

More available books at **www.hansebooks.com**

HEALTH

AND

EDUCATION

By CHARLES KINGSLEY

NEW EDITION

𝕷𝔬𝔫𝔡𝔬𝔫
MACMILLAN AND CO.
AND NEW YORK.
1887

(Originally published by Messrs. Daldy, Isbister & Co.   Reprinted by Messrs. Macmillan & Co., 1879, 1882, 1887.)

CONTENTS.

THE SCIENCE OF HEALTH.

WHETHER the British race is improving or degenerating?
What, if it seem probably degenerating, are the causes
of so great an evil? How they can be, if not destroyed,
at least arrested?—These are questions worthy the
attention, not of statesmen only and medical men,
but of every father and mother in these isles. I shall
say somewhat about them in this Essay; and say it in
a form which ought to be intelligible to fathers and
mothers of every class, from the highest to the lowest,
in hopes of convincing some of them at least that the
science of health, now so utterly neglected in our curriculum of so-called education, ought to be taught—the
rudiments of it at least—in every school, college, and
university.

We talk of our hardy forefathers; and rightly. But
they were hardy, just as the savage is usually hardy,
because none but the hardy lived. They may have
been able to say of themselves—as they do in a state

S   B

paper of 1515, now well known through the pages of
Mr. Froude—"What comyn folk of all the world may
compare with the comyns of England, in riches, freedom, liberty, welfare, and all prosperity? What comyn
folk is so mighty, and so strong in the felde, as the
comyns of England?" They may have been fed on
"great shins of beef," till they became, as Benvenuto
Cellini calls them, "the English wild beasts." But
they increased in numbers slowly, if at all, for centuries. Those terrible laws of natural selection, which
issue in "the survival of the fittest," cleared off the
less fit, in every generation, principally by infantile
disease, often by wholesale famine and pestilence; and
left, on the whole, only those of the strongest con-
stitutions to perpetuate a hardy, valiant, and enterprising race.

At last came a sudden and unprecedented change.
In the first years of the century, steam and commerce
produced an enormous increase in the population. Millions of fresh human beings found employment, married, brought up children who found employment in
their turn, and learnt to live more or less civilised
lives. An event, doubtless, for which God is to be
thanked. A quite new phase of humanity, bringing
with it new vices and new dangers: but bringing,
also, not merely new comforts, but new noblenesses, new
generosities, new conceptions of duty, and of how that

duty should be done. It is childish to regret the old times, when our soot-grimed manufacturing districts were green with lonely farms. To murmur at the transformation would be, I believe, to murmur at the will of Him without whom not a sparrow falls to the ground.

> "The old order changeth, yielding place to the new,
> And God fulfils himself in many ways,
> Lest one good custom should corrupt the world."

Our duty is, instead of longing for the good old custom, to take care of the good new custom, lest it should corrupt the world in like wise. And it may do so thus :—

The rapid increase of population during the first half of this century began at a moment when the British stock was specially exhausted; namely, about the end of the long French war. There may have been periods of exhaustion, at least in England, before that. There may have been one here, as there seems to have been on the Continent, after the Crusades; and another after the Wars of the Roses. There was certainly a period of severe exhaustion at the end of Elizabeth's reign, due both to the long Spanish and Irish wars and to the terrible endemics introduced from abroad; an exhaustion which may have caused, in part, the national weakness which hung upon us during the reign of the Stuarts. But after none of these did the survival of the less fit suddenly become more easy; or the discovery of steam power, and the acquisition of a colonial empire, create at once a fresh demand for human beings and a fresh supply of food for them. Britain, at the beginning of the nineteenth century, was in an altogether new social situation.

At the beginning of the great French war; and, indeed, ever since the beginning of the war with Spain in 1739—often snubbed as the "war about Jenkins's ear"—but which was, as I hold, one of the most just, as it was one of the most popular, of all our wars; after, too, the once famous "forty fine harvests" of the eighteenth century, the British people, from the gentleman who led to the soldier or sailor who followed, were one of the mightiest and most capable races which the world has ever seen, comparable best to the old Roman, at his mightiest and most capable period. That, at least, their works testify. They created—as far as man can be said to create anything—the British Empire. They won for us our colonies, our commerce, the mastery of the seas of all the world. But at what a cost—

> "Their bones are scattered far and wide,
> By mount, and stream, and sea."

Year after year, till the final triumph of Waterloo, not battle only, but worse destroyers than shot and shell—fatigue and disease—had been carrying off our stoutest,

ablest, healthiest young men, each of whom represented, alas! a maiden left unmarried at home, or
married, in default, to a less able man. The strongest
went to the war; each who fell left a weaklier man to
continue the race; while of those who did not fall, too
many returned with tainted and weakened constitu-
tions, to injure, it may be, generations yet unborn.
The middle classes, being mostly engaged in peaceful
pursuits, suffered less of this decimation of their finest
young men; and to that fact I attribute much of their
increasing preponderance, social, political, and intellectual, to this very day. One cannot walk the streets of any
of our great commercial cities without seeing plenty of
men, young and middle-aged, whose whole bearing and
stature shows that the manly vigour of our middle class
is anything but exhausted. In Liverpool, especially, I
have been much struck not only with the vigorous
countenance, but with the bodily size of the mercantile
men on 'Change. But it must be remembered always,
first, that these men are the very élite of their class;
the cleverest men; the men capable of doing most
work; and next, that they are, almost all of them, from
the great merchant who has his villa out of town, and
perhaps his moor in the Highlands, down to the sturdy
young volunteer who serves in the haberdasher's shop,
country-bred men; and that the question is, not what
they are like now, but what their children and grand-

children, especially the fine young volunteer's, will be like? And a very serious question I hold that to be; and for this reason.

War is, without doubt, the most hideous physical curse which fallen man inflicts upon himself; and for this simple reason, that it reverses the very laws of nature, and is more cruel even than pestilence. For instead of issuing in the survival of the fittest, it issues in the survival of the less fit: and therefore, if protracted, must deteriorate generations yet unborn. And yet a peace such as we now enjoy, prosperous, civilised, humane, is fraught, though to a less degree, with the very same ill effect.

In the first place, tens of thousands—Who knows it not?—lead sedentary and unwholesome lives, stooping, asphyxiated, employing as small a fraction of their bodies as of their minds. And all this in dwellings, workshops, what not?—the influences, the very atmosphere of which tend not to health, but to unhealth, and to drunkenness as a solace under the feeling of unhealth and depression. And that such a life must tell upon their offspring, and if their offspring grow up under similar circumstances, upon their offspring's offspring, till a whole population may become permanently degraded, who does not know? For who that walks through the by-streets of any great city does not see? Moreover, and this is one of the most fearful problems with which modern civilisation has to deal—we interfere with natural selection by our conscientious care of life, as surely as does war itself. If war kills the most fit to live, we save alive those who—looking at them from a merely physical point of view—are most fit to die. Everything which makes it more easy to live; every sanatory reform, prevention of pestilence, medical discovery, amelioration of climate, drainage of soil, improvement in dwelling-houses, workhouses, gaols; every reformatory school, every hospital, every cure of drunkenness, every influence, in short, which has—so I am told—increased the average length of life in these islands, by nearly one-third, since the first establishment of life insurances, one hundred and fifty years ago; every influence of this kind, I say, saves persons alive who would otherwise have died; and the great majority of these will be, even in surgical and zymotic cases, those of least resisting power; who are thus preserved to produce in time a still less powerful progeny.

Do I say that we ought not to save these people, if we can? God forbid. The weakly, the diseased, whether infant or adult, is here on earth; a British citizen; no more responsible for his own weakness than for his own existence. Society, that is, in plain English, we and our ancestors, are responsible for both; and we must fulfil the duty, and keep him in life; and, if we can, heal, strengthen, develop him to the utmost; and make the best of that which "fate and our own deservings" have given us to deal with. I do not speak of higher motives still; motives which to every minister of religion must be paramount and awful. I speak merely of physical and social motives, such as appeal to the conscience of every man—the instinct which bids every human-hearted man or woman to save life, alleviate pain, like Him who causes His sun to shine on the evil and on the good, and His rain to fall on the just and on the unjust.

But it is palpable, that in so doing we must, year by year, preserve a large percentage of weakly persons who, marrying freely in their own class, must produce weaklier children, and they weaklier children still. Must, did I say? There are those who are of opinion —and I, after watching and comparing the histories of many families, indeed, of every one with whom I have come in contact for now five-and-thirty years, in town and country, can only fear that their opinion is but too well founded on fact—that in the great majority of cases, in all classes whatsoever, the children are not equal to their parents, nor they, again, to their grand-parents of the beginning of the century; and that this degrading process goes on most surely, and most rapidly, in our large towns, and in proportion to the antiquity of those towns, and therefore in proportion to the number of generations during which the degrading influences have been at work.

This and cognate dangers have been felt more and more deeply, as the years have rolled on, by students of human society. To ward them off, theory after theory has been put on paper, especially in France, which deserve high praise for their ingenuity, less for their morality, and, I fear, still less for their common-sense. For the theorist in his closet is certain to ignore, as inconvenient to the construction of his Utopia, certain of those broad facts of human nature which every active parish priest, medical man, or poor-law guardian has to face every day of his life.

Society and British human nature are what they have become by the indirect influences of long ages, and we can no more reconstruct the one than we can change the other. We can no more mend men by theories than we can by coercion—to which, by the by, almost all these theorists look longingly as their final hope and mainstay. We must teach men to mend their own matters, of their own reason, and their own free-will. We must teach them that they are the arbiters of their own destinies; and, to a fearfully great degree, of their children's destinies after them. We must teach them not merely that they ought to be free, but that they are free, whether they know it or not, for good and for evil. And we must do that in this case, by teaching them sound practical science; the science of physiology as applied to health.   So, and so only, can we check—I do not say stop entirely—though I believe even that to be ideally possible; but at least check the process of degradation which I believe to be surely going on, not merely in these islands, but in every civilised country in the world, in proportion to its civilisation.

It is still a question whether science has fully discovered those laws of hereditary health, the disregard of which causes so many marriages disastrous to generations yet unborn.   But much valuable light has been thrown on this most mysterious and most important subject during the last few years.   That light—and I thank God for it—is widening and deepening rapidly.   And I doubt not that in a generation or two more enough will be known to be thrown into the shape of practical and proveable rules; and that, if not a public opinion, yet at least, what is more useful far, a wide-spread private opinion will grow up, especially among educated women, which will prevent many a tragedy and save many a life.

But, as to the laws of personal health : enough, and more than enough, is known already, to be applied safely and easily by any adults, however unlearned, to the preservation not only of their own health, but of that of their children.

The value of healthy habitations, of personal cleanliness, of pure air and pure water, of various kinds
of food, according as each tends to make bone, fat,
or muscle, provided only—provided only—that the
food be unadulterated; the value of various kinds of
clothing, and physical exercise, of a free and equal development of the brain-power, without undue overstrain
in any one direction; in one word, the method of producing, as far as possible, the mentem sanam in corpore
sano, and the wonderful and blessed effects of such
obedience to those laws of nature, which are nothing
but the good will of God expressed in facts—their
wonderful and blessed tendency, I say, to eliminate the
germs of hereditary disease, and to actually regenerate
the human system—all this is known; known as fully
and clearly as any human knowledge need be known;
it is written in dozens of popular books and pamphlets.
And why should this divine voice, which cries to man,
tending to sink into effeminate barbarism through his
own hasty and partial civilisation,—"It is not too late.
For your bodies, as for your spirits, there is an upward,
as well as a downward path. You, or if not you, at
least the children whom you have brought into the
world, for whom you toil, for whom you hoard, for
whom you pray, for whom you would give your lives,—
they still may be healthy, strong, it may be beautiful,
and have all the intellectual and social, as well as the

physical advantages, which health, strength, and beauty give."—Ah, why is this divine voice now, as of old, Wisdom crying in the streets, and no man regarding her ? I appeal to women, who are initiated, as we men can never be, into the stern mysteries of pain, and sorrow, and self-sacrifice;—they who bring forth children, weep over children, slave for children, and, if they have none of their own, then slave, with the holy instinct of the sexless bee, for the children of others— Let them say, shall this thing be ?

Let my readers pardon me if I seem to write too earnestly. That I speak neither more nor less than the truth, every medical man knows full well. Not only as a very humble student of physiology, but as a parish priest of thirty years' standing, I have seen so much unnecessary misery; and I have in other cases seen similar misery so simply avoided; that the sense of the vastness of the evil is intensified by my sense of the easiness of the cure.

Why, then—to come to practical suggestions—should there not be opened in every great town in these realms a public school of health? It might connect itself with—I hold that it should form an integral part of— some existing educational institute. But it should at least give practical lectures, for fees small enough to put them within the reach of any respectable man or woman, however poor. I cannot but hope that such schools of health, if opened in the great manufacturing towns of England and Scotland, and, indeed, in such an Irish town as Belfast, would obtain pupils in plenty, and pupils who would thoroughly profit by what they hear. The people of these towns are, most of them, specially accustomed by their own trades to the application of scientific laws. To them, therefore, the application of any fresh physical laws to a fresh set of facts, would have nothing strange in it. They have already something of that inductive habit of mind which is the groundwork of all rational understanding or action. They would not turn the deaf and contemptuous ear with which the savage and the superstitious receive the revelation of nature's mysteries. Why should not, with so hopeful an audience, the experiment be tried far and wide, of giving lectures on health, as supplementary to those lectures on animal physiology which are, I am happy to say, becoming more and more common? Why should not people be taught—they are already being taught at Birmingham—something about the tissues of the body, their structure and uses, the circulation of the blood, respiration, chemical changes in the air respired, amount breathed, digestion, nature of food, absorption, secretion, structure of the nervous system,—in fact, be taught something of how their own bodies are made and how they work? Teaching of this kind ought to, and will, in some more civilised age and country, be held a necessary element in the school-course of every child, just as necessary as reading, writing, and arithmetic; for it is after all the most necessary branch of that "technical education" of which we hear so much just now, namely, the technic, or art, of keeping oneself alive and well.

But we can hardly stop there. After we have taught the condition of health, we must teach also the condition of disease; of those diseases specially which tend to lessen wholesale the health of townsfolk, exposed to an artificial mode of life. Surely young men and women should be taught something of the causes of zymotic disease, and of scrofula, consumption, rickets, dipsomania, cerebral derangement, and such like. They should be shown the practical value of pure air, pure water, unadulterated food, sweet and dry dwellings. Is there one of them, man or woman, who would not be the safer and happier, and the more useful to his or her neighbours, if they had acquired some sound notions about those questions of drainage on which their own lives and the lives of their children may every day depend? I say—women as well as men. I should have said women rather than men. For it is the women who have the ordering of the household, the bringing up of the children; the women who bide at home, while the men are away, it may be at the other end of the earth.

And if any say, as they have a right to say—"But these are subjects which can hardly be taught to young women in public lectures;" I rejoin,—Of course not, unless they are taught by women,—by women, of course, duly educated and legally qualified. Let such teach to women, what every woman ought to know, and what her parents will very properly object to her hearing from almost any man. This is one of the main reasons why I have, for twenty years past, advocated the training of women for the medical profession; and one which countervails, in my mind, all possible objections to such a movement. And now, thank God, I am seeing the common sense of Great Britain, and indeed of every civilised nation, gradually coming round to that which seemed to me, when I first conceived of it, a dream too chimerical to be cherished save in secret —the restoring woman to her natural share in that sacred office of healer, which she held in the Middle Ages, and from which she was thrust out during the sixteenth century.

I am most happy to see, for instance, that the National Health Society,* which I earnestly recommend to the attention of my readers, announces a "Course of Lectures for Ladies on Elementary Physiology and Hygiene, by Miss Chessar," to which I am also most happy to see, governesses are admitted at half-fees. Alas!

* 9, Adam Street, Adelphi, London.

how much misery, disease, and even death, might have
been prevented, had governesses been taught such
matters thirty years ago, I, for one, know too well.
May the day soon come when there will be educated
women enough to give such lectures throughout these
realms, to rich as well as poor,—for the rich, strange
to say, need them often as much as the poor do,—and
that we may live to see, in every great town, health
classes for women as well as for men, sending forth
year by year more young women and young men
taught, not only to take care of themselves and of their
families, but to exercise moral influence over their
fellow-citizens, as champions in the battle against dirt
and drunkenness, disease and death.

There may be those who would answer—or rather,
there would certainly have been those who would have
so answered thirty years ago, before the so-called
materialism of advanced science had taught us some
practical wisdom about education, and reminded people
that they have bodies as well as minds and souls—
"You say, we are likely to grow weaklier, unhealthier.
And if it were so, what matter?   Mind makes the man,
not body.   We do not want our children to be stupid
giants and bravos; but clever, able, highly educated,
however weakly Providence or the laws of nature may
have chosen to make them.   Let them overstrain their
brains a little; let them contract their chests, and

injure their digestion and their eyesight, by sitting at
desks, poring over books. Intellect is what we want.
Intellect makes money. Intellect makes the world. We
would rather see our son a genius than an athlete."
Well: and so would I. But what if intellect alone
does not even make money, save as Messrs. Dodson &
Fogg, Sampson Brass, and Montagu Tigg were wont
to make it, unless backed by an able, enduring, healthy
physique, such as I have seen, almost without exception,
in those successful men of business whom I have had
the honour and the pleasure of knowing? What if
intellect, or what is now called intellect, did not make
the world, or the smallest wheel or cog of it? What
if, for want of obeying the laws of nature, parents bred
up neither a genius nor an athlete, but only an incapable unhappy personage, with a huge upright forehead,
like that of a Byzantine Greek, filled with some sort
of pap instead of brains, and tempted alternately to
fanaticism and strong drink? We must, in the great
majority of cases have the corpus sanem if we want
the mentem sanem; and healthy bodies are the only
trustworthy organs for healthy minds. Which is cause
and which is effect, I shall not stay to debate here.
But wherever we find a population generally weakly,
stunted, scrofulous, we find in them a corresponding
type of brain, which cannot be trusted to do good work;

which is capable more or less of madness, whether solitary or epidemic. It may be very active; it may be very quick at catching at new and grand ideas—all the more quick, perhaps, on account of its own secret *malaise* and self-discontent: but it will be irritable, spasmodic, hysterical. It will be apt to mistake capacity of talk for capacity of action, excitement for earnestness, virulence for force, and, too often, cruelty for justice. It will lose manful independence, individuality, originality; and when men act, they will act from the consciousness of personal weakness, like sheep rushing over a hedge, leaning against each other, exhorting each other to be brave, and swaying about in mobs and masses. These were the intellectual weaknesses which, as I read history, followed on physical degradation in Imperial Rome, in Alexandria, in Byzantium. Have we not seen them reappear, under fearful forms, in Paris but the other day?

I do not blame; I do not judge. My theory, which I hold, and shall hold, to be fairly founded on a wide induction, forbids me to blame and to judge: because it tells me that these defects are mainly physical; that those who exhibit them are mainly to be pitied, as victims of the sins or ignorance of their forefathers. But it tells me too, that those who, professing to be educated men, and therefore bound to know better, treat these physical phenomena as spiritual, healthy, and praiseworthy; who even exasperate them, that they may make capital out of the weaknesses of fallen man, are the most contemptible and yet the most dangerous of public enemies, let them cloak their quackery under whatsoever patriotic, or scientific, or even sacred words.

There are those again honest, kindly, sensible, practical men, many of them; men whom I have no wish to offend; whom I had rather ask to teach me some of their own experience and common sense, which has learned to discern, like good statesmen, not only what ought to be done, but what can be done—there are those, I say, who would sooner see this whole question let alone. Their feeling, as far as I can analyse it, seems to be, that the evils of which I have been complaining, are on the whole inevitable: or, if not, that we can mend so very little of them, that it is wisest to leave them alone altogether, lest, like certain sewers, "the more you stir them, the more they smell." They fear lest we should unsettle the minds of the many for whom these evils will never be mended; lest we make them discontented; discontented with their houses, their occupations, their food, their whole social arrangements; and all in vain.

I should answer, in all courtesy and humility—for I sympathise deeply with such men and women, and respect them deeply likewise—But are not people dis-

contented already, from the lowest to the highest?
And ought a man, in such a piecemeal, foolish, greedy,
sinful world as this is, and always has been, to be anything but discontented? If he thinks that things are
going all right, must he not have a most beggarly
conception of what going right means? And if things
are not going right, can it be anything but good for
him to see that they are not going right? Can truth
and fact harm any human being? I shall not believe
so, as long as I have a Bible wherein to believe. For
my part, I should like to make every man, woman, and
child whom I meet discontented with themselves, even
as I am discontented with myself. I should like to
awaken in them, about their physical, their intellectual,
their moral condition, that divine discontent which is
the parent, first of upward aspiration and then of self-
control, thought, effort to fulfil that aspiration even in
part. For to be discontented with the divine discontent, and to be ashamed with the noble shame, is the
very germ and first upgrowth of all virtue. Men begin
at first, as boys begin when they grumble at their
school and their schoolmasters, to lay the blame on
others; to be discontented with their circumstances—
the things which stand around them; and to cry, "Oh
that I had this!" "Oh that I had that!" But that
way no deliverance lies. That discontent only ends
in revolt and rebellion, social or political; and that,

again, still in the same worship of circumstances—but this time desperate—which ends, let it disguise itself under what fine names it will, in what the old Greeks called a tyranny; in which—as in the Spanish republics of America, and in France more than once—all have become the voluntary slaves of one man, because each man fancies that the one man can improve his circumstances for him.

But the wise man will learn, like Epictetus the heroic slave, the slave of Epaphroditus, Nero's minion —and in what baser and uglier circumstances could human being find himself?—to find out the secret of being truly free; namely, to be discontented with no man and no thing save himself. To say not—" Oh that I had this and that ! " but " Oh that I were this and that ! " Then, by God's help—and that heroic slave, heathen though he was, believed and trusted in God's help—" I will make myself that which God has shown me that I ought to be and can be."

Ten thousand a-year, or ten million a-year, as Epictetus saw full well, cannot mend that vulgar discontent with circumstances, which he had felt—and who with more right?—and conquered, and despised. For that is the discontent of children, wanting always more holidays and more sweets. But I wish my readers to have, and to cherish, the discontent of men and women.

Therefore I would make men and women discontented, with the divine and wholesome discontent, at their own physical frame, and at that of their children. I would accustom their eyes to those precious heirlooms of the human race, the statues of the old Greeks; to their tender grandeur, their chaste healthfulness, their unconscious, because perfect, might: and say— There; these are tokens to you, and to all generations yet unborn, of what man could be once; of what he can be again if he will obey those laws of nature which are the voice of God. I would make them discontented with the ugliness and closeness of their dwellings; I would make them discontented with the fashion of their garments, and still more just now the women, of all ranks, with the fashion of theirs; and with everything around them which they have the power of improving, if it be at all ungraceful, superfluous, tawdry, ridiculous, unwholesome. I would make them discontented with what they call their education, and say to them—You call the three Royal R's education? They are not education: no more is the knowledge which would enable you to take the highest prizes given by the Society of Arts, or any other body. They are not education: they are only instruction; a necessary groundwork, in an age like this, for making practical use of your education: but not the education itself.

And if they asked me, What then education meant?

I should point them, first, I think, to noble old Lilly's noble old 'Euphues,' of three hundred years ago, and ask them to consider what it says about education, and especially this passage concerning that mere knowledge which is nowadays strangely miscalled education. " There are two principal and peculiar gifts in the nature of man, knowledge and reason. The one " —that is reason—" commandeth, and the other "—that is knowledge—" obeyeth. These things neither the whirling wheel of fortune can change, nor the deceitful cavillings of worldlings separate, neither sickness abate, nor age abolish.". And next I should point them to those pages in Mr. Gladstone's 'Juventus Mundi,' where he describes the ideal training of a Greek youth in Homer's days ; and say,—There : that is an education fit for a really civilised man, even though he never saw a book in his life ; the full, proportionate, harmonious educing—that is, bringing out and developing —of all the faculties of his body, mind, and heart, till he becomes at once a reverent yet a self-assured, a graceful and yet a valiant, an able and yet an eloquent personage.

And if any should say to me—"But what has this to do with science ? Homer's Greeks knew no science;"" I should rejoin—But they had, pre-eminently above all ancient races which we know, the scientific instinct; the teachableness and modesty; the clear eye and

quick ear; the hearty reverence for fact and nature,
and for the human body, and mind, and spirit; for
human nature, in a word, in its completeness, as the
highest fact upon this earth.   Therefore they became
in after years, not only the great colonisers and the
great civilisers of the old world—the most practical
people, I hold, which the world ever saw; but the
parents of all sound physics as well as of all sound
metaphysics.   Their very religion, in spite of its im-
perfections, helped forward their education, not in
spite of, but by means of, that anthropomorphism
which we sometimes too hastily decry.   As Mr. Gladstone says in a passage which I must quote at length—
"As regarded all other functions of our nature, outside the domain of the life to Godward—all those functions which are summed up in what St. Paul calls the
flesh and the mind, the psychic and bodily life, the
tendency of the system was to exalt the human element, by proposing a model of beauty, strength, and
wisdom, in all their combinations, so elevated that
the effort to attain them required a continual upward
strain.   It made divinity attainable; and thus it effec-
tually directed the thought and aim of man

‘ Along the line of limitless desires.’

Such a scheme of religion, though failing grossly in
the government of the passions, and in upholding the

standard of moral duties, tended powerfully to produce a lofty self-respect, and a large, free, and varied conception of humanity. It incorporated itself in schemes of notable discipline for mind and body, indeed of a lifelong education; and these habits of mind and action had their marked results (to omit many other greatnesses) in a philosophy, literature, and art, which remain to this day unrivalled or unsurpassed."

So much those old Greek did for their own education, without science and without Christianity. We who have both: what might we not do, if we would be true to our advantages, and to ourselves?

THE TWO BREATHS.

A LECTURE DELIVERED AT WINCHESTER, MAY 31, 1869.

———◦◦———

LADIES,—I have been honoured by a second invitation to address you here, from the lady to whose public spirit the establishment of these lectures is due. I dare not refuse it: because it gives me an opportunity of speaking on a matter, knowledge and ignorance about which may seriously affect your health and happiness, and that of the children with whom you may have to do. I must apologize if I say many things which are well known to many persons in this room: they ought to be well known to all; and it is generally best to assume total ignorance in one's hearers, and to begin from the beginning.

I shall try to be as simple as possible; to trouble you as little as possible with scientific terms; to be practical; and at the same time, if possible, interesting.

I should wish to call this lecture "The Two Breaths:" not merely " The Breath ; " and for this reason : every time you breathe, you breathe two different breaths; you take in one, you give out another. The composition of those two breaths is different. Their effects are different. The breath which has been breathed out must not be breathed in again. To tell you why it must not would lead me into anatomical details, not quite in place here as yet : though the day will come, I trust, when every woman entrusted with the care of children will be expected to know something about them. But this I may say—Those who habitually take in fresh breath will probably grow up large, strong, ruddy, cheerful, active, clear-headed, fit for their work. Those who habitually take in the breath which has been breathed out by themselves, or any other living creature, will certainly grow up, if they grow up at all, small, weak, pale, nervous, depressed, unfit for work, and tempted continually to resort to stimulants, and become drunkards.

If you want to see how different the breath breathed out is from the breath taken in, you have only to try a somewhat cruel experiment, but one which people too often try upon themselves, their children, and their work-people. If you take any small animal with lungs like your own—a mouse, for instance—and force it to breathe no air but what you have breathed already; if you put it in a close box, and while you take in breath from the outer air, send out your breath through a tube, into

that box, the animal will soon faint; if you go on long
with this process, it will die.

Take a second instance, which I beg to press most
seriously on the notice of mothers, governesses, and
nurses: If you allow the child to get into the habit of
sleeping with its head under the bed-clothes, and thereby
breathing its own breath over and over again, that child
will assuredly grow pale, weak, and ill. Medical men
have cases on record of scrofula appearing in children
previously healthy, which could only be accounted for
from this habit, and which ceased when the habit
stopped. Let me again entreat your attention to this
undoubted fact.

Take another instance, which is only too common:
If you are in a crowded room, with plenty of fire and
lights and company, doors and windows all shut tight,
how often you feel faint—so faint, that you may require
smelling-salts or some other stimulant. The cause of
your faintness is just the same as that of the mouse's
fainting in the box: you and your friends, and, as I
shall show you presently, the fire and the candles likewise, having been all breathing each other's breaths,
over and over again, till the air has become unfit to
support life. You are doing your best to enact over
again the Highland tragedy, of which Sir James Simpson
tells in his lectures to the working-classes of Edinburgh,
when at a Christmas meeting thirty-six persons danced

all night in a small room with a low ceiling, keeping the doors and windows shut. The atmosphere of the room was noxious beyond description; and the effect was, that seven of the party were soon after seized with typhus fever, of which two died. You are inflicting on yourselves the torments of the poor dog, who is kept at the Grotto del Cane, near Naples, to be stupified, for the amusement of visitors, by the carbonic acid gas of the Grotto, and brought to life again by being dragged into the fresh air; nay, you are inflicting upon yourselves the torments of the famous Black Hole of Calcutta; and, if there was no chimney in the room, by which some fresh air could enter, the candles would soon burn blue—as they do, you know, when ghosts appear; your brains become disturbed; and you yourselves run the risk of becoming ghosts, and the candles of actually going out.

Of this last fact there is no doubt; for if, instead of putting a mouse into the box, you will put a lighted candle, and breathe into the tube, as before, however gently, you will in a short time put the candle out.

Now, how is this? First, what is the difference between the breath you take in and the breath you give out? And next, why has it a similar effect on animal life and a lighted candle?

The difference is this. The breath which you take in is, or ought to be, pure air, composed, on the whole, of oxygen and nitrogen, with a minute portion of carbonic acid.

The breath which you give out is an impure air, to which has been added, among other matters which will not support life, an excess of carbonic acid.

That this is the fact you can prove for yourselves by a simple experiment. Get a little lime water at the chemist's, and breathe into it through a glass tube; your breath will at once make the lime-water milky. The carbonic acid of your breath has laid hold of the lime, and made it visible as white carbonate of lime—in plain English, as common chalk.

Now, I do not wish, as I said, to load your memories with scientific terms: but I beseech you to remember at least these two—oxygen gas and carbonic acid gas; and to remember that, as surely as oxygen feeds the fire of life, so surely does carbonic acid put it out.

I say, "the fire of life." In that expression lies the answer to our second question: Why does our breath produce a similar effect upon the mouse and the lighted candle? Every one of us is, as it were, a living fire. Were we not, how could we be always warmer than the air outside us? There is a process going on perpetually in each of us, similar to that by which coals are burnt in the fire, oil in a lamp, wax in a candle, and the earth itself in a volcano. To keep each of those fires alight, oxygen is needed; and the products of combustion, as they are called, are more or less the same in each case—carbonic acid and steam.

These facts justify the expression I just made use of—which may have seemed to some of you fantastical—that the fire and the candles in the crowded room were breathing the same breath as you were. It is but too true. An average fire in the grate requires, to keep it burning, as much oxygen as several human beings do; each candle or lamp must have its share of oxygen likewise, and that a very considerable one; and an average gas-burner—pray attend to this, you who live in rooms lighted with gas—consumes as much oxygen as several candles. All alike are making carbonic acid. The carbonic acid of the fire happily escapes up the chimney in the smoke: but the carbonic acid from the human beings and the candles remains to poison the room, unless it be ventilated.

Now, I think you may understand one of the simplest, and yet most terrible, cases of want of ventilation—death by the fumes of charcoal. A human being shut up in a room, of which every crack is closed, with a pan of burning charcoal, falls asleep, never to wake again. His inward fire is competing with the fire of the charcoal for the oxygen of the room; both are making carbonic acid out of it: but the charcoal, being the stronger of the two, gets all the oxygen to itself, and leaves the human being nothing to inhale but the carbonic acid which it has made. The human being, being the weaker, dies first: but the charcoal dies also. When it has exhausted all the oxygen of the room, it cools, goes out, and is found in the morning half-consumed beside its victim. If you put a giant or an elephant, I should conceive, into that room, instead of a human being, the case would be reversed for a time: the elephant would put out the burning charcoal by the carbonic acid from his mighty lungs; and then, when he had exhausted all the air in the room, die likewise of his own carbonic acid.

Now, I think, we may see what ventilation means, and why it is needed.

Ventilation means simply letting out the foul air, and letting in the fresh air; letting out the air which has been breathed by men or by candles, and letting in the air which has not. To understand how to do that, we must remember a most simple chemical law, that a gas as it is warmed expands, and therefore becomes lighter; as it cools, it contracts, and becomes heavier.

Now the carbonic acid in the breath which comes out of our mouth is warm, lighter than the air, and rises to the ceiling; and therefore in any unventilated room full of people, there is a layer of foul air along the ceiling. You might soon test that for yourselves, if you could mount a ladder and put your heads there aloft. You do test it for yourselves when you sit in the galleries of churches and theatres, where the air is palpably more foul, and therefore more injurious, than down below.

Where, again, work-people are employed in a crowded house of many storeys, the health of those who work on the upper floors always suffers most.

In the old monkey-house of the Zoological Gardens, when the cages were on the old plan, tier upon tier, the poor little fellows in the uppermost tier—so I have been told—always died first of the monkey's constitutional complaint, consumption, simply from breathing the warm breath of their friends below. But since the cages have been altered, and made to range side by side from top to bottom, consumption—I understand—has vastly diminished among them.

The first question in ventilation, therefore, is to get this carbonic acid safe out of the room, while it is warm and light and close to the ceiling; for if you do not, this happens—The carbonic acid gas cools and becomes heavier; for carbonic acid, at the same temperature as common air, is so much heavier than common air, that you may actually—if you are handy enough—turn it from one vessel to another, and pour out for your enemy a glass of invisible poison. So down to the floor this heavy carbonic acid comes, and lies along it, just as it lies often in the bottom of old wells, or old

D

brewers' vats, as a stratum of poison, killing occasionally the men who descend into it. Hence, as foolish a practice as I know is that of sleeping on the floor; for towards the small hours, when the room gets cold, the sleeper on the floor is breathing carbonic acid.

And here one word to those ladies who interest themselves with the poor. The poor are too apt in times of distress to pawn their bedsteads and keep their beds. Never, if you have influence, let that happen. Keep the bedstead, whatever else may go, to save the sleeper from the carbonic acid on the floor.

How, then, shall we get rid of the foul air at the top of the room? After all that has been written and tried on ventilation, I know no simpler method than putting into the chimney one of Arnott's ventilators, which may be bought and fixed for a few shillings; always remembering that it must be fixed into the chimney as near the ceiling as possible. I can speak of these ventilators from twenty-five years' experience. Living in a house with low ceilings, liable to become overcharged with carbonic acid, which produces sleepiness in the evening, I have found that these ventilators keep the air fresh and pure; and I consider the presence of one of these ventilators in a room more valuable than three or four feet additional height of ceiling. I have found, too, that their working proves how necessary they are, from this simple fact :—You would suppose that, as the ventilator opens freely into the chimney, the smoke would be blown down through it in high winds, and blacken the ceiling : but this is just what does not happen. If the ventilator be at all properly poised, so as to shut with a violent gust of wind, it will at all other moments keep itself permanently open ; proving thereby that there is an up-draught of heated air continually escaping from the ceiling up the chimney. Another very simple method of ventilation is employed in those excellent cottages which Her Majesty has built for her labourers round Windsor. Over each door a sheet of perforated zinc, some 18 inches square, is fixed ; allowing the foul air to escape into the passage ; and in the ceiling of the passage a similar sheet of zinc, allowing it to escape into the roof. Fresh air, meanwhile, should be obtained from outside, by piercing the windows, or otherwise. And here let me give one hint to all builders of houses. If possible, let bedroom windows open at the top as well as at the bottom.

Let me impress the necessity of using some such contrivances, not only on parents and educators, but on those who employ work-people, and above all on those who employ young women in shops or in work-rooms. What their condition may be in this city I know not ; but most painful it has been to me in other places, when passing through warehouses or work-rooms, to see the pale, sodden, and, as the French would say "etiolated" countenances of the girls who were passing the greater part of the day in them; and painful, also, to breathe an atmosphere of which habit had, alas! made them unconscious, but which to one coming out of the open air was altogether noxious, and shocking also; for it was fostering the seeds of death, not only in the present but in future generations.

Why should this be? Every one will agree that good ventilation is necessary in a hospital, because people cannot get well without fresh air. Do they not see that by the same reasoning good ventilation is necessary everywhere, because people cannot remain well without fresh air? Let me entreat those who employ women in work-rooms, if they have no time to read through such books as Dr. Andrew Combe's 'Physiology applied to Health and Education,' and Madame de Wahl's 'Practical Hints on the Moral, Mental, and Physical Training of Girls,' to procure certain tracts published by Messrs. Jarrold, Paternoster Row, for the Ladies' Sanitary Association; especially one which bears on this subject, 'The Black-Hole in our own Bedrooms;' Dr. Lankester's 'School Manual of Health;' or a manual on ventilation, published by the Metropolitan Working Classes Association for the Improvement of Public Health.

I look forward—I say it openly—to some period of

higher civilisation, when the Acts of Parliament for the ventilation of factories and workshops shall be largely extended, and made far more stringent; when officers of public health shall be empowered to enforce the ventilation of every room in which persons are employed for hire: and empowered also to demand a proper system of ventilation for every new house, whether in country or in town. To that, I believe, we must come: but I had sooner far see these improvements carried out, as befits the citizens of a free country, in the spirit of the Gospel rather than in that of the Law; carried out, not compulsorily and from fear of fines, but voluntarily, from a sense of duty, honour, and humanity. I appeal, therefore, to the good feeling of all whom it may concern, whether the health of those whom they employ, and therefore the supply of fresh air which they absolutely need, are not matters for which they are not, more or less, responsible to their country and their God.

And if any excellent person of the old school should answer me—" Why make all this fuss about ventilation? Our forefathers got on very well without it "—I must answer that, begging their pardons, our ancestors did nothing of the kind. Our ancestors got on usually very ill in these matters: and when they got on well, it was because they had good ventilation in spite of themselves.

First. They got on very ill.   To quote a few remarkable instances of longevity, or to tell me that men
were larger and stronger on the average in old times, is
to yield to the old fallacy of fancying that savages were
peculiarly healthy, because those who were seen were
active and strong.   The simple answer is, that the
strong alone survived, while the majority died from
the severity of the training.   Savages do not increase
in number; and our ancestors increased but very slowly
for many centuries.   I am not going to disgust my
audience with statistics of disease: but knowing something, as I happen to do, of the social state and of the
health of the Middle and Elizabethan Ages, I have no
hesitation in saying that the average of disease and
death was far greater then than it is now.   Epidemics
of many kinds, typhus, ague, plague—all diseases which
were caused more or less by bad air—devastated this
land and Europe in those days with a horrible intensity,
to which even the choleras of our times are mild.   The
back streets, the hospitals, the gaols, the barracks, the
camps—every place in which any large number of
persons congregated, were so many nests of pestilence,
engendered by uncleanliness, which defiled alike the
water which was drunk and the air which was breathed;
and as a single fact, of which the tables of insurance
companies assure us, the average of human life in
England has increased twenty-five per cent. since the

reign of George I., owing simply to our more rational and cleanly habits of life.

But secondly, I said that when our ancestors got on well, they did so because they got ventilation in spite of themselves. Luckily for them, their houses were ill-built; their doors and windows would not shut. They had lattice-windowed houses, too; to live in one of which, as I can testify from long experience, is as thoroughly ventilating as living in a lantern with the horn broken out. It was because their houses were full of draughts, and still more, in the early middle age, because they had no glass, and stopped out the air only by a shutter at night, that they sought for shelter rather than for fresh air, of which they sometimes had too much; and, to escape the wind, built their houses in holes, such as that in which the old city of Winchester stands. Shelter, I believe, as much as the desire to be near fish in Lent, and to occupy the rich alluvium of the valleys, made the monks of Old England choose the river-banks for the sites of their abbeys. They made a mistake therein, which, like most mistakes, did not go unpunished. These low situations, especially while the forests were yet thick on the hills around, were the perennial haunts of fever and ague, produced by subtle vegetable poisons, carried in the carbonic acid given off by rotting vegetation. So there, again, they fell in with man's old enemy—bad air.

Still, as long as the doors and windows did not shut, some free circulation of air remained. But now, our doors and windows shut only too tight. We have plate-glass instead of lattices; and we have replaced the draughty and smoky, but really wholesome open chimney, with its wide corners and settles, by narrow registers, and even by stoves. We have done all we can, in fact, to seal ourselves up hermetically from the outer air, and to breathe our own breaths over and over again; and we pay the penalty of it in a thousand ways unknown to our ancestors, through whose rooms all the winds of heavens whistled, and who were glad enough to shelter themselves from draughts in the sitting-room by the high screen round the fire, and in the sleeping-room by the thick curtains of the four-post bedstead, which is now rapidly disappearing before a higher civilisation. We therefore absolutely require to make for ourselves the very ventilation from which our ancestors tried to escape.

But, ladies, there is an old and true proverb, that you may bring a horse to the water, but you cannot make him drink. And in like wise it is too true, that you may bring people to the fresh air, but you cannot make them breathe it. Their own folly, or the folly of their parents and educators, prevents their lungs being duly filled and duly emptied. Therefore, the blood is not duly oxygenated, and the whole system goes wrong.

Paleness, weakness, consumption, scrofula, and too many other ailments, are the consequences of ill-filled lungs. For without well-filled lungs, robust health is impossible.

And if any one shall answer—"We do not want robust health so much as intellectual attainment. The mortal body, being the lower organ, must take its chance, and be even sacrificed, if need be, to the higher organ— the immortal mind : "—To such I reply, You cannot do it. The laws of nature, which are the express will of God, laugh such attempts to scorn. Every organ of the body is formed out of the blood; and if the blood be vitiated, every organ suffers in proportion to its delicacy; and the brain, being the most delicate and highly specialised of all organs, suffers most of all and soonest of all, as every one knows who has tried to work his brain when his digestion was the least out of order. Nay, the very morals will suffer. From ill-filled lungs, which signify ill-repaired blood, arise year by year an amount not merely of disease, but of folly, temper, laziness, intemperance, madness, and, let me tell you fairly, crime—the sum of which will never be known till that great day when men shall be called to account for all deeds done in the body, whether they be good or evil.

I must refer you on this subject again to Andrew Combe's ' Physiology,' especially chapters iv. and vii.;

and also to chapter x. of Madame de Wahl's excellent book. I will only say this shortly, that the three most common causes of ill-filled lungs, in children and in young ladies, are stillness, silence, and stays.

First, stillness; a sedentary life, and want of exercise. A girl is kept for hours sitting on a form writing or reading, to do which she must lean forward; and if her schoolmistress cruelly attempts to make her sit upright, and thereby keep the spine in an attitude for which Nature did not intend it, she is thereby doing her best to bring on that disease, so fearfully common in girls' schools, lateral curvature of the spine. But practically the girl will stoop forward. And what happens? The lower ribs are pressed into the body, thereby displacing more or less something inside. The diaphragm in the meantime, which is the very bellows of the lungs, remains loose; the lungs are never properly filled or emptied; and an excess of carbonic acid accumulates at the bottom of them. What follows? Frequent sighing to get rid of it; heaviness of head; depression of the whole nervous system under the influence of the poison of the lungs; and when the poor child gets up from her weary work, what is the first thing she probably does? She lifts up her chest, stretches, yawns, and breathes deeply—Nature's voice, Nature's instinctive cure, which is probably regarded as ungraceful, as what is called "lolling" is. As if sitting upright was not an attitude in itself essentially ungraceful, and such as no artist would care to draw. As if "lolling," which means putting the body in the attitude of the most perfect ease compatible with a fully expanded chest, was not in itself essentially graceful, and to be seen in every reposing figure in Greek bas-reliefs and vases; graceful, and like all graceful actions, healthful at the same time. The only tolerably wholesome attitude of repose, which I see allowed in average school-rooms, is lying on the back on the floor, or on a sloping board, in which case the lungs must be fully expanded. But even so, a pillow, or some equivalent, ought to be placed under the small of the back: or the spine will be strained at its very weakest point.

I now go on to the second mistake—enforced silence. Moderate reading aloud is good: but where there is any tendency to irritability of throat or lungs, too much moderation cannot be used. You may as well try to cure a diseased lung by working it, as to cure a lame horse by galloping him. But where the breathing organs are of average health, let it be said once and for all, that children and young people cannot make too much noise. The parents who cannot bear the noise of their children have no right to have brought them into the world. The schoolmistress who enforces silence on her pupils is committing—unintentionally no doubt, but still committing—an offence against reason, worthy only of a convent. Every shout, every burst of laughter, every song—nay, in the case of infants, as physiologists well know, every moderate fit of crying—conduces to health, by rapidly filling and emptying the lung, and changing the blood more rapidly from black to red, that is, from death to life. Andrew Combe tells a story of a large charity school, in which the young girls were, for the sake of their health, shut up in the hall and school-room during play hours, from November till March, and no romping or noise allowed. The natural consequences were, the great majority of them fell ill; and I am afraid that a great deal of illness has been from time to time contracted in certain school-rooms, simply through this one cause of enforced silence. Some cause or other there must be for the amount of ill-health and weakliness which prevails especially among girls of the middle classes in towns, who have not, poor things, the opportunities which richer girls have, of keeping themselves in strong health by riding, skating, archery—that last quite an admirable exercise for the chest and lungs, and far preferable to croquet, which involves too much unwholesome stooping.—Even playing at ball, if milliners and shop-girls had room to indulge in one after their sedentary work, might bring fresh spirits to many a heart, and fresh colour to many a cheek.

I spoke just now of the Greeks. I suppose you will

all allow that the Greeks were, as far as we know, the most beautiful race which the world ever saw. Every educated man knows that they were also the cleverest of all races; and, next to his Bible, thanks God for Greek literature.

Now, these people had made physical as well as intellectual education a science as well as a study. Their women practised graceful, and in some cases even athletic, exercises. They developed, by a free and healthy life, those figures which remain everlasting and unapproachable models of human beauty: but—to come to my third point—they wore no stays. The first mention of stays that I have ever found is in the letters of dear old Synesius, Bishop of Cyrene, on the Greek coast of Africa, about four hundred years after the Christian era. He tells us how, when he was shipwrecked on a remote part of the coast, and he and the rest of the passengers were starving on cockles and limpets, there was among them a slave girl out of the far East, who had a pinched wasp-waist, such as you may see on the old Hindoo sculptures, and such as you may see in any street in a British town. And when the Greek ladies of the neighbourhood found her out, they sent for her from house to house, to behold, with astonishment and laughter, this new and prodigious waist, with which it seemed to them it was impossible for a human being to breathe or live; and they petted the poor girl, and fed her, as they might a dwarf or a giantess, till she got quite fat and comfortable, while her owners had not enough to eat. So strange and ridiculous seemed our present fashion to the descendants of those who, centuries before, had imagined, because they had seen living and moving, those glorious statues which we pretend to admire, but refuse to imitate.

It seems to me that a few centuries hence, when mankind has learnt to fear God more, and therefore to obey more strictly those laws of nature and of science which are the will of God—it seems to me, I say, that in those days the present fashion of tight lacing will be looked back upon as a contemptible and barbarous superstition, denoting a very low level of civilisation in the peoples which have practised it. That for generations past women should have been in the habit—not to please men, who do not care about the matter as a point of beauty—but simply to vie with each other in obedience to something called fashion—that they should, I say, have been in the habit of deliberately crushing that part of the body which should be specially left free, contracting and displacing their lungs, their heart, and all the most vital and important organs, and entailing thereby disease, not only on themselves but on their children after them; that for forty years past physicians should have been telling them of the folly of what they have been doing: and that they should, as yet, in the

great majority of cases, not only turn a deaf ear to all
warnings, but actually deny the offence, of which one
glance of the physician or the sculptor, who know what
shape the human body ought to be, brings them in
guilty: this, I say, is an instance of—what shall I call
it?—which deserves at once the lash, not merely of the
satirist, but of any theologian who really believes that
God made the physical universe. Let me, I pray you,
appeal to your common sense for a moment. When any
one chooses a horse or a dog, whether for strength, foı
speed, or for any other useful purpose, the first thing
almost to be looked at is the girth round the ribs;
the room for heart and lungs. Exactly in proportion
to that will be the animal's general healthiness, power
of endurance, and value in many other ways. If you
will look at eminent lawyers and famous orators, who
have attained a healthy old age, you will see that in
every case they are men, like the late Lord Palmerston,
and others whom I could mention, of remarkable size,
not merely in the upper, but in the lower part of the
chest; men who had, therefore, a peculiar power of
using the diaphragm to fill and to clear the lungs, and
therefore to oxygenate the blood of the whole body.
Now, it is just these lower ribs, across which the diaphragm is stretched like the head of a drum, which
stays contract to a minimum. If you advised owners
of horses and hounds to put their horses or their hounds

into stays, and lace them up tight, in order to increase their beauty, you would receive, I doubt not, a very courteous, but certainly a very decided, refusal to do that which would spoil not merely the animals them-selves, but the whole stud or the whole kennel for years to come. And if you advised an orator to put him-self into tight stays, he, no doubt, again would give a courteous answer; but he would reply—if he was a really educated man—that to comply with your request would involve his giving up public work, under the probable penalty of being dead within the twelve-month.

And how much work of every kind, intellectual as well as physical, is spoiled or hindered; how many deaths occur from consumption and other complaints which are the result of this habit of tight lacing, is known partly to the medical men, who lift up their voices in vain, and known fully to Him who will not interfere with the least of His own physical laws to save human beings from the consequences of their own wilful folly.

And now—to end this lecture with more pleasing thoughts—What becomes of this breath which passes from your lips? Is it merely harmful; merely waste? God forbid! God has forbidden that anything should be merely harmful or merely waste in this so wise and well-made world. The carbonic acid which passes from your lips at every breath—ay, even that which oozes from the volcano crater when the eruption is past—is a precious boon to thousands of things of which you have daily need. Indeed there is a sort of hint at physical truth in the old fairy tale of the girl, from whose lips, as she spoke, fell pearls and diamonds; for the carbonic acid of your breath may help hereafter to make the pure carbonate of lime of a pearl, or the still purer carbon of a diamond. Nay, it may go—in such a world of transformations do we live—to make atoms of coal strata, which shall lie buried for ages beneath deep seas, shall be upheaved in continents which are yet unborn, and there be burnt for the use of a future race of men, and resolved into their original elements. Coal, wise men tell us, is on the whole breath and sunlight; the breath of living creatures who have lived in the vast swamps and forests of some primæval world, and the sunlight which transmuted that breath into the leaves and stems of trees, magically locked up for ages in that black stone, to become, when it is burnt at last, light and carbonic acid, as it was at first. For though you must not breathe your breath again, you may at least eat your breath, if you will allow the sun to transmute it for you into vegetables; or you may enjoy its fragrance and its colour in the shape of a lily or a rose. When you walk in a sunlit garden, every word you speak, every breath you breathe, is feeding the plants

E

and flowers around. The delicate surface of the green leaves absorbs the carbonic acid, and parts it into its elements, retaining the carbon to make woody fibre, and courteously returning you the oxygen to mingle with the fresh air, and be inhaled by your lungs once more. Thus do you feed the plants; just as the plants feed you; while the great life-giving sun feeds both; and the geranium standing in the sick child's window does not merely rejoice his eye and mind by its beauty and freshness, but repays honestly the trouble spent on it; absorbing the breath which the child needs not, and giving to him the breath which he needs.

So are the services of all things constituted according to a Divine and wonderful order, and knit together in mutual dependence and mutual helpfulness.—A fact to be remembered with hope and comfort; but also with awe and fear. For as in that which is above nature, so in nature itself; he that breaks one physical law is guilty of all. The whole universe, as it were, takes up arms against him; and all nature, with her numberless and unseen powers, is ready to avenge herself on him, and on his children after him, he knows not when nor where. He, on the other hand, who obeys the laws of nature with his whole heart and mind, will find all things working together to him for good. He is at peace with the physical universe. He is helped and

befriended alike by the sun above his head and the
dust beneath his feet: because he is obeying the will
and mind of Him who made sun, and dust, and all
things; and who has given them a law which cannot
be broken.

THE TREE OF KNOWLEDGE.

THE more I have contemplated that ancient story of the Fall, the more it has seemed to me within the range of probability, and even of experience. It must have happened somewhere for the first time; for it has happened only too many times since. It has happened, as far as I can ascertain, in every race, and every age, and every grade of civilisation. It is happening round us now in every region of the globe. Always and everywhere, it seems to me, have poor human beings been tempted to eat of some "tree of knowledge," that they may be, even for an hour, as gods; wise, but with a false wisdom; careless, but with a frantic carelessness; and happy, but with a happiness which, when the excitement is past, leaves too often—as with that hapless pair in Eden—depression, shame, and fear. Everywhere, and in all ages, as far as I can ascertain, has man been inventing stimulants and narcotics to supply that want of vitality of which he is so painfully aware;

and has asked nature, and not God, to clear the dull brain, and comfort the weary spirit.

This has been, and will be perhaps for many a century to come, almost the most fearful failing of this poor, exceptional, over-organised, diseased, and truly fallen being called man, who is in doubt daily whether he be a god or an ape; and in trying wildly to become the former, ends but too often in becoming the latter.

For man, whether savage or civilised, feels, and has felt in every age, that there is something wrong with him. He usually confesses this fact—as is to be expected—of his fellow-men, rather than of himself; and shows his sense that there is something wrong with them by complaining of, hating, and killing them. But he cannot always conceal from himself the fact that he, too, is wrong, as well as they; and as he will not usually kill himself, he tries wild ways to make himself at least feel—if not to be—somewhat "better." Philosophers may bid him be content; and tell him that he is what he ought to be, and what nature has made him. But he cares nothing for the philosophers. He knows, usually, that he is not what he ought to be; that he carries about with him, in most cases, a body more or less diseased and decrepit, incapable of doing all the work which he feels that he himself could do, or expressing all the emotions which he himself longs to express; a dull brain and dull senses, which cramp the eager infinity within him; as—so Goethe once said with pity—the horse's single hoof cramps the fine intelligence and generosity of his nature, and forbids him even to grasp an object, like the more stupid cat, and baser monkey. And man has a self, too, within, from which he longs too often to escape, as from a household ghost; who pulls out, at unfortunately rude and unwelcome hours, the ledger of memory. And so when the tempter—be he who he may—says to him " Take this, and you will 'feel better '—Take this, and you shall be as gods, knowing good and evil: " then, if the temptation was, as the old story says, too much for man while healthy and unfallen, what must it be for his unhealthy and fallen children ?

In vain we say to man—

> " 'Tis life, not death, for which you pant;
> 'Tis life, whereof your nerves are scant;
> More life, and fuller, that you want."

And your tree of knowledge is not the tree of life: it is, in every case, the tree of death; of decrepitude, madness, misery. He prefers the voice of the tempter —" Thou shalt not surely die." Nay, he will say at last,—" Better be as gods awhile, and die: than be the crawling, insufficient thing I am; and live."

He—did I say? Alas! I must say she likewise. The sacred story is only too true to fact, when it represents the woman as falling, not merely at the same time as the man, but before the man. Only let us remember that it represents the woman as tempted; tempted, seemingly, by a rational being, of lower race, and yet of superior cunning; who must, therefore, have fallen before the woman. Who or what the being was, who is called the Serpent in our translation of Genesis, it is not for me to say. We have absolutely, I think, no facts from which to judge; and Rabbinical traditions need trouble no man much. But I fancy that a missionary, preaching on this story to Negroes; telling them plainly that the "Serpent" meant the first Obeah man; and then comparing the experiences of that hapless pair in Eden, with their own after certain orgies not yet extinct in Africa and elsewhere, would be only too well understood: so well, indeed, that he might run some risk of eating himself, not of the tree of life, but of that of death. The sorcerer or sorceress tempting the woman; and then the woman tempting the man; this seems to be, certainly among savage peoples, and, alas! too often among civilised peoples also, the usual course of the world-wide tragedy.

But—paradoxical as it may seem—the woman's yielding before the man is not altogether to her dishonour, as those old monks used to allege who hated, and too often tortured, the sex whom they could not enjoy. It is not to the woman's dishonour, if she felt, before her husband, higher aspirations than those after mere animal pleasure. To be as gods, knowing good and evil, is a vain and foolish, but not a base and brutal, wish. She proved herself thereby—though at an awful cost—a woman, and not an animal. And indeed the woman's more delicate organisation, her more vivid emotions, her more voluble fancy, as well as her mere physical weakness and weariness, have been to her, in all ages, a special source of temptation; which it is to her honour that she has resisted so much better than the physically stronger, and therefore more culpable, man.

As for what the tree of knowledge was, there really is no need for us to waste our time in guessing. If it was not one plant, then it was another. It may have been something which has long since perished off the earth. It may have been—as some learned men have guessed — the sacred Soma, or Homa, of the early Brahmin race; and that may have been a still existing narcotic species of Asclepias. It certainly was not the vine. The language of the Hebrew Scripture concerning it, and the sacred use to which it is consecrated in the Gospels, forbid that notion utterly; at least to those who know enough of antiquity to pass by, with a smile, the theory that the wines mentioned in Scripture were not intoxicating. And yet—as a fresh corroboration of what I am trying to say—how fearfully has that noble gift to man been abused for the same end as a hundred other vegetable products, ever since those mythic days when Dionusos brought the vine from the far East, amid troops of human Mænads and half-human Satyrs; and the Bacchæ tore Pentheus in pieces on Cithæron, for daring to intrude upon their sacred rites; and since those historic days, too, when, less than two hundred years before the Christian era, the Bacchic rites spread from Southern Italy into Etruria, and thence to the matrons of Rome; and under the guidance of Pœnia Annia, a Campanian lady, took at last shapes of which no man must speak, but which had to be put down with terrible but just severity, by the Consuls and the Senate.

But it matters little, I say, what this same tree of knowledge was. Was every vine on earth destroyed to-morrow, and every vegetable also from which alcohol is now distilled, man would soon discover something else wherewith to satisfy the insatiate craving. Has he not done so already? Has not almost every people had its tree of knowledge, often more deadly than any distilled liquor, from the absinthe of the cultivated Frenchman, and the opium of the cultivated Chinese, down to the bush-poisons wherewith the tropic sorcerer initiates his dupes into the knowledge of good and evil, and the fungus from which the Samoiede extracts in autumn a few days of brutal happiness, before the setting in of the long six months' night? God grant that modern science may not bring to light fresh substitutes for alcohol, opium, and the rest; and give the white races, in that state of effeminate and godless quasi-civilisation which I sometimes fear is creeping upon them, fresh means of destroying themselves delicately and pleasantly off the face of the earth.

It is said by some that drunkenness is on the increase in this island. I have no trusty proof of it : but I can believe it possible; for every cause of drunkenness seems on the increase. Overwork of body and mind; circumstances which depress health; temptation to drink, and drink again, at every corner of the streets; and finally, money, and ever more money, in the hands of uneducated people, who have not the desire, and too often not the means, of spending it in any save the lowest pleasures. These, it seems to me, are the true causes of drunkenness, increasing or not. And if we wish to become a more temperate nation, we must lessen them, if we cannot eradicate them.

First, overwork. We all live too fast, and work too hard. "All things are full of labour, man cannot utter it." In the heavy struggle for existence which goes on all around us, each man is tasked more and more—if he be really worth buying and using—to the utmost of his powers all day long. The weak have to compete on equal terms with the strong; and crave, in consequence, for artificial strength. How we shall stop that I know

not, while every man is "making haste to be rich, and
piercing himself through with many sorrows, and falling
into foolish and hurtful lusts, which drown men in
destruction and perdition." How we shall stop that, I
say, I know not. The old prophet may have been right
when he said, "Surely it is not of the Lord that the
people shall labour in the very fire, and weary themselves for very vanity;" and in some juster, wiser, more
sober system of society—somewhat more like the Kingdom of The Father come on earth—it may be that poor
human beings will not need to toil so hard, and to keep
themselves up to their work by stimulants, but will
have time to sit down, and look around them, and think
of God, and of God's quiet universe, with something of
quiet in themselves; something of rational leisure, and
manful sobriety of mind, as well as of body.

But it seems to me also, that in such a state of society,
when—as it was once well put—"every one has stopped
running about like rats:"—that those who work hard,
whether with muscle or with brain, would not be surrounded, as now, with every circumstance which
tempts toward drink; by every circumstance which
depresses the vital energies, and leaves them an easy
prey to pestilence itself; by bad light, bad air, bad
food, bad water, bad smells, bad occupations, which
weaken the muscles, cramp the chest, disorder the
digestion. Let any rational man, fresh from the coun-

try—in which I presume God, having made it, meant all men, more or less, to live—go through the back streets of any city, or through whole districts of the "black countries" of England: and then ask himself —Is it the will of God that His human children should live and toil in such dens, such deserts, such dark places of the earth? Let him ask himself —Can they live and toil there without contracting a probably diseased habit of body; without contracting a certainly dull, weary, sordid habit of mind, which craves for any pleasure, however brutal, to escape from its own stupidity and emptiness? When I run through, by rail, certain parts of the iron-producing country— streets of furnaces, collieries, slag heaps, mud, slop, brick house-rows, smoke, dirt—and that is all; and when I am told, whether truly or falsely, that the main thing which the well-paid and well-fed men of those abominable wastes care for is—good fighting-dogs: I can only answer, that I am not surprised.

I say—as I have said elsewhere, and shall do my best to say again—that the craving for drink and narcotics, especially that engendered in our great cities, is not a disease, but a symptom of disease; of a far deeper disease than any which drunkenness can produce; namely, of the growing degeneracy of a population striving in vain by stimulants and narcotics to fight against those slow poisons with which our greedy barbarism, miscalled civilisation, has surrounded them from the cradle to the grave. I may be answered that the old German, Angle, Dane, drank heavily. I know it: but why did they drink, save for the same reason that the fenman drank, and his wife took opium, at least till the fens were drained? why but to keep off the depressing effects of the malaria of swamps and new clearings, which told on them—who always settled in the lowest grounds—in the shape of fever and ague? Here it may be answered again, that stimulants have been, during the memory of man, the destruction of the Red Indian race in America. I reply boldly, that I do not believe it. There is evidence enough in Jacques Cartier's 'Voyages to the Rivers of Canada;' and evidence more than enough in Strachey's 'Travaile in Virginia'—to quote only two authorities out of many —to prove that the Red Indians, when the white man first met with them, were, in North and South alike, a diseased, decaying, and, as all their traditions confess, decreasing race. Such a race would naturally crave for "the water of life," the "usque-bagh," or whisky, as we have contracted the old name now. But I should have thought that the white man, by introducing among these poor creatures iron, fire-arms, blankets, and above all horses wherewith to follow the buffalo-herds which they could never follow on foot, must have done ten times more towards keeping them alive, than he has done towards destroying them by giving them the chance of a week's drunkenness twice a year, when they came in to his forts to sell the skins which, without his gifts, they would never have got.

Such a race would, of course, if wanting vitality, crave for stimulants. But if the stimulants, and not the original want of vitality, combined with morals utterly detestable, and worthy only of the gallows—and here I know what I say, and dare not tell what I know, from eye-witnesses—have been the cause of the Red Indians' extinction: then how is it, let me ask, that the Irishman and the Scotsman have, often to their great harm, been drinking as much whisky—and usually very bad whisky—not merely twice a year, but as often as they could get it, during the whole "iron age;" and, for aught any one can tell, during the "bronze age," and the "stone age " before that: and yet are still the most healthy, able, valiant, and prolific races in Europe? Had they drunk less whisky they would, doubtless, have been more healthy, able, valiant, and perhaps even more prolific, than they are now. They show no sign, however, as yet, of going the way of the Red Indian.

But if the craving for stimulants and narcotics is a token of deficient vitality: then the deadliest foe of that craving, and all its miserable results, is surely the Sanatory Reformer; the man who preaches, and—as far as ignorance and vested interests will allow him, procures—for the masses, pure air, pure sunlight, pure water, pure dwelling-houses, pure food. Not merely every fresh drinking-fountain: but every fresh public bath and wash-house, every fresh open space, every fresh growing tree, every fresh open window, every fresh flower in that window—each of these is so much, as the old Persians would have said, conquered for Ormuzd, the god of light and life, out of the dominion of Ahriman, the king of darkness and of death; so much taken from the causes of drunkenness and disease, and added to the causes of sobriety and health.

Meanwhile one thing is clear: that if this present barbarism and anarchy of covetousness, miscalled modern civilisation, were tamed and drilled into something more like a Kingdom of God on earth: then we should not see the reckless and needless multiplication of liquor shops, which disgraces this country now.

As a single instance: in one country parish of nine hundred inhabitants, in which the population has increased only one-ninth in the last fifty years, there are now practically eight public-houses, where fifty years ago there were but two. One, that is, for every hundred and ten—or rather, omitting children, farmers, shopkeepers, gentlemen, and their households, one for every fifty of the inhabitants. In the face of the allurements, often of the basest kind, which these dens offer, the clergyman and the schoolmaster struggle in vain to keep up night-schools and young men's clubs, and to inculcate habits of providence.

The young labourers over a great part of the south and east, at least of England,—though never so well off, for several generations, as they are now—are growing up thriftless, shiftless; inferior, it seems to me, to their grandfathers in everything, save that they can usually read and write, and their grandfathers could not; and that they wear smart cheap cloth clothes, instead of their grandfathers' smock-frocks.

And if it be so in the country: how must it be in towns? There must come a thorough change in the present licensing system, in spite of all the "pressure" which certain powerful vested interests may bring to bear on governments. And it is the duty of every good citizen, who cares for his countrymen, and for their children after them, to help in bringing about that change as speedily as possible.

Again: I said just now that a probable cause of increasing drunkenness was the increasing material prosperity of thousands who knew no recreation beyond low animal pleasure. If I am right—and I believe that I am right—I must urge on those who wish drunkenness to decrease, the necessity of providing more, and more refined recreation for the people.

Men drink, and women too, remember, not merely

to supply exhaustion; not merely to drive away care: but often simply to drive away dulness. They have nothing to do save to think over what they have done in the day, or what they expect to do to-morrow; and they escape from that dreary round of business thought, in liquor or narcotics. There are still those, by no means of the hand-working class, but absorbed all day by business, who drink heavily at night in their own comfortable homes, simply to recreate their over-burdened minds. Such cases, doubtless, are far less common than they were fifty years ago: but why? Is not the decrease of drinking among the richer classes certainly due to the increased refinement and variety of their tastes and occupations? In cultivating the æsthetic side of man's nature; in engaging him with the beautiful, the pure, the wonderful, the truly natural; with painting, poetry, music, horticulture, physical science—in all this lies recreation, in the true and literal sense of that word, namely, the re-creating and mending of the exhausted mind and feelings, such as no rational man will now neglect, either for himself, his children, or his workpeople.

But how little of all this is open to the masses, all should know but too well. How little opportunity the average hand-worker, or his wife, has of eating of any tree of knowledge, save of the very basest kind, is but too palpable. We are mending, thank God, in this

F

respect.   Free libraries and museums have sprung up
of late in other cities beside London.   God's blessing
rest upon them all.   And the Crystal Palace, and still
later, the Bethnal Green Museum, have been, I believe,
of far more use than many average sermons and lectures from many average orators.

But are we not still far behind the old Greeks, and
the Romans of the Empire likewise, in the amount of
amusement and instruction, and even of shelter, which
we provide for the people?   Recollect the—to me—dis-
graceful fact; that there is not, as far as I am aware,
throughout the whole of London, a single portico or
other covered place, in which the people can take
refuge during a shower: and this in the climate of
England!   Where they do take refuge on a wet day
the publican knows but too well; as he knows also ·
where thousands of the lower classes, simply for want
of any other place to be in, save their own sordid
dwellings, spend as much as they are permitted of the
Sabbath day.   Let us put down " Sunday drinking" by
all means, if we can.   But let us remember that by
closing the public-houses on Sunday, we prevent no
man or woman from carrying home as much poison as
they choose on Saturday night, to brutalise themselves
therewith, perhaps for eight-and-forty hours.   And let
us see—in the name of Him who said that He had made
the Sabbath for man, and not man for the Sabbath—

let us see, I say, if we cannot do something to prevent the townsman's Sabbath being, not a day of rest, but a day of mere idleness; the day of most temptation, because of most dulness, of the whole seven.

And here, perhaps, some sweet soul may look up reprovingly and say—He talks of rest. Does he forget, and would he have the working man forget, that all these outward palliatives will never touch the seat of the disease, the unrest of the soul within? Does he forget, and would he have the working man forget, who it was who said—who only has the right to say—" Come unto Me, all ye who are weary and heavy laden, and I will give you rest"? Ah no, sweet soul. I know your words are true. I know that what we all want is inward rest; rest of heart and brain; the calm, strong, self-contained, self-denying character; which needs no stimulants, for it has no fits of depression; which needs no narcotics, for it has no fits of excitement; which needs no ascetic restraints, for it is strong enough to use God's gifts without abusing them; the character, in a word, which is truly temperate, not in drink or food merely, but in all desires, thoughts, and actions; freed from the wild lusts and ambitions to which that old Adam yielded, and, seeking for light and life by means forbidden, found thereby disease and death. Yes; I know that; and know, too, that that rest is found, only where you have already found it.

And yet: in such a world as this; governed by a Being who has made sunshine, and flowers, and green grass, and the song of birds, and happy human smiles; and who would educate by them—if we would let Him —His human children from the cradle to the grave; in such a world as this, will you grudge any particle of that education, even any harmless substitute for it, to those spirits in prison whose surroundings too often tempt them, from the cradle to the grave, to fancy that the world is composed of bricks and iron, and governed by inspectors and policemen? Preach to those spirits in prison, as you know far better than we parsons how to preach; but let them have besides some glimpses of the splendid fact, that outside their prison-house is a world which God, not man, has made; wherein grows everywhere that tree of knowledge, which is likewise the tree of life; and that they have a right to some small share of its beauty, and its wonder, and its rest, for their own health of soul and body, and for the health of their children after them.

NAUSICAA IN LONDON:

OR, THE LOWER EDUCATION OF WOMAN.

FRESH from the Marbles of the British Museum, I went my way through London streets. My brain was still full of fair and grand forms; the forms of men and women whose every limb and attitude betokened perfect health, and grace, and power, and a, self-possession and self-restraint so habitual and complete that it had become unconscious, and undistinguishable from the native freedom of the savage. For I had been up and down the corridors of those Greek sculptures, which remain as a perpetual sermon to rich and poor, amid our artificial, unwholesome, and it may be decaying pseudo-civilisation; saying with looks more expressive than all words—Such men and women can be; for such they have been; and such you may be yet, if you will use that science of which you too often only boast. Above all, I had been pondering over the awful and yet tender beauty of the maiden figures from the

Parthenon and its kindred temples. And these, or such
as these, I thought to myself, were the sisters of the
men who fought at Marathon and Salamis; the mothers
of many a man among the ten thousand whom Xeno-
phon led back from Babylon to the Black Sea shore;
the ancestresses of many a man who conquered the
East in Alexander's host, and fought with Porus in the
far Punjab. And were these women mere dolls? These
men mere gladiators? Were they not the parents of
philosophy, science, poetry, the plastic arts? We talk
of education now. Are we more educated than were
the ancient Greeks? Do we know anything about
education, physical, intellectual, or æsthetic, and I may
say moral likewise—religious education, of course, in
our sense of the word, they had none—but do we know
anything about education of which they have not taught
us at least the rudiments? Are there not some branches
of education which they perfected, once and for ever;
leaving us northern barbarians to follow, or else not to
follow, their example? To produce health, that is,
harmony and sympathy, proportion and grace, in every
faculty of mind and body—that was their notion of
education. To produce that, the text-book of their
childhood was the poetry of Homer, and not of—— But
I am treading on dangerous ground. It was for this
that the seafaring Greek lad was taught to find his
ideal in Ulysses; while his sister at home found hers, it

may be, in Nausicaa. It was for this, that when perhaps the most complete and exquisite of all the Greeks,
Sophocles the good, beloved by gods and men, represented on the Athenian stage his drama of Nausicaa, and,
as usual, could not—for he had no voice—himself take a
speaking part, he was content to do one thing in which
he specially excelled; and dressed and masked as a girl,
to play at ball amid the chorus of Nausicaa's maidens.

That drama of Nausicaa is lost; and if I dare say so
of any play of Sophocles', I scarce regret it. It is well,
perhaps, that we have no second conception of the
scene, to interfere with the simplicity, so grand, and
yet so tender, of Homer's idyllic episode.

Nausicaa, it must be remembered, is the daughter of
a king. But not of a king in the exclusive modern
European or old Eastern sense. Her father, Alcinous,
is simply "primus inter pares" among a community of
merchants, who are called "kings" likewise; and
Mayor for life—so to speak—of a new trading city, a
nascent Genoa or Venice, on the shore of the Mediterranean. But the girl Nausicaa, as she sleeps in her
"carved chamber," is "like the immortals in form and
face;" and two handmaidens who sleep on each side of
the polished door "have beauty from the Graces."

To her there enters, in the shape of some maiden
friend, none less than Pallas Athené herself, intent on
saving worthily her favourite, the shipwrecked Ulysses:

and bids her in a dream go forth—and wash the
clothes.*

> " Nausicaa, wherefore doth thy mother bear
>   Child so forgetful ?   This long time doth rest,
>   Like lumber in the house, much raiment fair.
>   Soon must thou wed, and be thyself well-drest,
>   And find thy bridegroom raiment of the best.
>   These are the things whence good repute is born,
>   And praises that make glad a parent's breast.
>   Come, let us both go washing with the morn ;
> So shalt thou have clothes becoming to be worn.
>
> " Know that thy maidenhood is not for long,
>   Whom the Phœacian chiefs already woo,
>   Lords of the land whence thou thyself art sprung.
>   Soon as the shining dawn comes forth anow,
>   For wain and mules thy noble father sue,
>   Which to the place of washing shall convey
>   Girdles and shawls and rugs of splendid hue.
>   This for thyself were better than essay
> Thither to walk : the place is distant a long way."

Startled by her dream, Nausicaa awakes, and goes to
find her parents—

> " One by the hearth sat, with the maids around,
>   And on the skeins of yarn, sea-purpled, spent
>   Her morning toil.   Him to the council bound,
> Called by the honoured kings, just going forth she found."

And calling him, as she might now, "Pappa phile,"
Dear Papa, asks for the mule waggon : but it is her
father's and her five brothers' clothes she fain would
wash,—

> " Ashamed to name her marriage to her father dear."

---

* I quote from the translation of the late lamented Philip Stanhope
Worsley, of Corpus Christi College, Oxford.

But he understood all—and she goes forth in the mule
waggon, with the clothes, after her mother has put in
"a chest of all kinds of delicate food, and meat, and wine
in a goatskin;" and last but not least, the indispensable
cruse of oil for anointing after the bath, to which both
Jews, Greeks, and Romans owed so much health and
beauty. And then we read in the simple verse of a poet
too refined, like the rest of his race, to see anything mean
or ridiculous in that which was not ugly and unnatural,
how she and her maids got into the "polished waggon,"
"with good wheels," and she "took the whip and the
studded reins," and "beat them till they started;" and
how the mules "rattled" away, and "pulled against
each other," till

> " When they came to the fair flowing river
> Which feeds good lavatories all the year,
> Fitted to cleanse all sullied robes soever,
> They from the wain the mules unharnessed there,
> And chased them free, to crop their juicy fare
> By the swift river, on the margin green;
> Then to the waters dashed the clothes they bare
> And in the stream-filled trenches stamped them clean.

> " Which, having washed and cleansed, they spread before
> The sunbeams, on the beach, where most did lie
> Thick pebbles, by the sea-wave washed ashore.
> So, having left them in the heat to dry,
> They to the bath went down, and by-and-by,
> Rubbed with rich oil, their midday meal essay,
> Conched in green turf, the river rolling nigh.
> Then, throwing off their veils, at ball they play,
> While the white-armed Nausicaa leads the choral lay."

The mere beauty of this scene all will feel, who have the sense of beauty in them. Yet it is not on that aspect which I wish to dwell, but on its healthfulness. Exercise is taken, in measured time, to the sound of song, as a duty almost, as well as an amusement. For this game of ball, which is here mentioned for the first time in human literature, nearly three thousand years ago, was held by the Greeks and by the Romans after them, to be an almost necessary part of a liberal education ; principally, doubtless, from the development which it produced in the upper half of the body, not merely to the arms, but to the chest, by raising and expanding the ribs, and to all the muscles of the torso, whether perpendicular or oblique. The elasticity and grace which it was believed to give were so much prized, that a room for ball-play, and a teacher of the art, were integral parts of every gymnasium ; and the Athenians went so far as to bestow on one famous ball-player, Aristonicus of Carystia, a statue and the rights of citizenship. The rough and hardy young Spartans, when passing from boyhood into manhood, received the title of ball-players, seemingly from the game which it was then their special duty to learn. In the case of Nausicaa and her maidens, the game would just bring into their right places all that is liable to be contracted and weakened in women, so many of whose occupations must needs be sedentary and stooping ; while the song which accompanied the game at once filled the lungs regularly and rhythmically, and prevented violent motion, or unseemly attitude. We, the civilised, need physiologists to remind us of these simple facts, and even then do not act on them. Those old half-barbarous Greeks had found them out for themselves, and, moreover, acted on them.

But fair Nausicaa must have been—some will say— surely a mere child of nature, and an uncultivated person ?

So far from it, that her whole demeanour and speech show culture of the very highest sort, full of " sweetness and light."—Intelligent and fearless, quick to perceive the bearings of her strange and sudden adventure, quick to perceive the character of Ulysses, quick to answer his lofty and refined pleading by words as lofty and refined, and pious withal;—for it is she who speaks to her handmaids the once so famous words:

> " Strangers and poor men all are sent from Zeus;
> And alms, though small, are sweet."

Clear of intellect, prompt of action, modest of demeanour, shrinking from the slightest breath of scandal; while she is not ashamed, when Ulysses, bathed and dressed, looks himself again, to whisper to her maidens her wish that the Gods might send her such a spouse.—This is Nausicaa as Homer draws her ; and as many a scholar and poet since Homer has accepted

her for the ideal of noble maidenhood. I ask my
readers to study for themselves her interview with
Ulysses, in Mr. Worsley's translation, or rather in the
grand simplicity of the original Greek,* and judge
whether Nausicaa is not as perfect a lady as the poet
who imagined her—or, it may be, drew her from life—
must have been a perfect gentleman; both complete
in those "manners" which, says the old proverb,
"make the man:" but which are the woman herself;
because with her—who acts more by emotion than by
calculation—manners are the outward and visible
tokens of her inward and spiritual grace, or disgrace;
and flow instinctively, whether good or bad, from the
instincts of her inner nature.

True, Nausicaa could neither read nor write. No
more, most probably, could the author of the Odyssey.
No more, for that matter, could Abraham, Isaac, and
Jacob, though they were plainly, both in mind and
manners, most highly-cultivated men. Reading and
writing, of course, have now become necessaries of
humanity; and are to be given to every human being,
that he may start fair in the race of life. But I am
not aware that Greek women improved much, either in
manners, morals, or happiness, by acquiring them in
after centuries. A wise man would sooner see his

* Odyssey, book vi. 127-315; vol. i. pp. 143-150 of Mr. Worsley's
translation.

daughter a Nausicaa than a Sappho, an Aspasia, a Cleopatra, or even an Hypatia.

Full of such thoughts, I went through London streets, among the Nausicaas of the present day; the girls of the period; the daughters and hereafter mothers of our future rulers, the great Demos or commercial middle class of the greatest mercantile city in the world: and noted what I had noted with fear and sorrow, many a day, for many a year; a type, and an increasing type, of young women who certainly had not had the "advantages," "educational" and other, of that Greek Nausicaa of old.

Of course, in such a city as London, to which the best of everything, physical and other, gravitates, I could not but pass, now and then, beautiful persons, who made me proud of those "grandes Anglaises aux joues rouges," whom the Parisiennes ridicule—and envy. But I could not help suspecting that their looks showed them to be either country-bred, or born of country parents; and this suspicion was strengthened by the fact, that when compared with their mothers, the mother's physique was, in the majority of cases, superior to the daughters'. Painful it was, to one accustomed to the ruddy well-grown peasant girl, stalwart, even when, as often, squat and plain, to remark the exceedingly small size of the average young woman; by which I do not mean mere want of height—that is

a little matter—but want of breadth likewise; a general
want of those large frames, which indicate usually a
power of keeping strong and healthy not merely the
muscles, but the brain itself.

Poor little things.   I passed hundreds—I pass hundreds every day—trying to hide their littleness by the
nasty mass of false hair—or what does duty for it;
and by the ugly and useless hat which is stuck upon
it, making the head thereby look ridiculously large and
heavy; and by the high heels on which they totter
onward, having forgotten, or never learnt, the simple
art of walking; their bodies tilted forward in that
ungraceful attitude which is called—why that name of
all others?—a "Grecian bend;" seemingly kept on
their feet, and kept together at all, in that strange
attitude, by tight stays which prevented all graceful
and healthy motion of the hips or sides; their raiment,
meanwhile, being purposely misshapen in this direction and in that, to hide—it must be presumed—
deficiencies of form.   If that chignon and those heels
had been taken off, the figure which would have remained would have been that too often of a puny girl
of sixteen.   And yet there was no doubt that these
women were not only full grown, but some of them,
alas! wives and mothers.

Poor little things.—And this they have gained by so-
called civilisation: the power of aping the "fashions"

by which the worn-out Parisienne hides her own personal defects; and of making themselves, by innate want of that taste which the Parisienne possesses, only the cause of something like a sneer from many a cultivated man; and of something like a sneer, too, from yonder gipsy woman who passes by, with bold bright face, and swinging hip, and footstep stately and elastic; far better dressed, according to all true canons of taste, than most town-girls; and thanking her fate that she and her "Rom" are no house-dwellers and gaslight-sightseers, but fatten on free air upon the open moor.

But the face which is beneath that chignon and that hat? Well—it is sometimes pretty: but how seldom handsome, which is a higher quality by far. It is not, strange to say, a well-fed face. Plenty of money, and perhaps too much, is spent on those fine clothes. It had been better, to judge from the complexion, if some of that money had been spent in solid wholesome food. She looks as if she lived—as she too often does, I hear —on tea and bread-and-butter, or rather on bread with the minimum of butter. For as the want of bone indicates a deficiency of phosphatic food, so does the want of flesh about the cheeks indicate a deficiency of hydrocarbon. Poor little Nausicaa:—that is not her fault. Our boasted civilisation has not even taught her what to eat, as it certainly has not increased her appetite; and she knows not—what every country fellow knows—that without plenty of butter and other fatty matters, she is not likely to keep even warm. Better to eat nasty fat bacon now, than to supply the want of it some few years hence by nastier cod-liver oil. But there is no one yet to tell her that, and a dozen other equally simple facts, for her own sake, and for the sake of that coming Demos which she is to bring into the world; a Demos which, if we can only keep it healthy in body and brain, has before it so splendid a future : but which, if body and brain degrade beneath the influence of modern barbarism, is but too likely to follow the Demos of ancient Byzantium, or of modern Paris.

Ay, but her intellect. She is so clever, and she reads so much, and she is going to be taught to read so much more.

Ah, well—there was once a science called physiognomy. The Greeks, from what I can learn, knew more of it than any people since : though the Italian painters and sculptors must have known much; far more than we. In a more scientific civilisation there will be such a science once more : but its laws, though still in the empiric stage, are not altogether forgotten by some. Little children have often a fine and clear instinct of them. Many cultivated and experienced women have a fine and clear instinct of them likewise. And some

such would tell us that there is intellect in plenty in
the modern Nausicaa: but not of the quality which
they desire for their country's future good. Self-con-
sciousness, eagerness, volubility, petulance, in countenance, in gesture, and in voice—which last is too often
most harsh and artificial, the breath being sent forth
through the closed teeth, and almost entirely at the
corners of the mouth—and, with all this, a weariness
often about the wrinkling forehead and the drooping
lids;—all these, which are growing too common, not
among the Demos only, nor only in the towns, are
signs, they think, of the unrest of unhealth, physical,
intellectual, spiritual. At least they are as different as
two types of physiognomy in the same race can be,
from the expression both of face and gesture, in those
old Greek sculptures, and in the old Italian painters;
and, it must be said, in the portraits of Reynolds, and
Gainsborough, Copley, and Romney. Not such, one
thinks, must have been the mothers of Britain during
the latter half of the last century and the beginning of
the present; when their sons, at times, were holding
half the world at bay.

And if Nausicaa has become such in town: what is
she when she goes to the seaside, not to wash the
clothes in fresh-water, but herself in salt—the very
salt-water, laden with decaying organisms, from which,
though not polluted further by a dozen sewers, Ulysses

G

had to cleanse himself, anointing, too, with oil, ere he
was fit to appear in the company of Nausicaa of Greece?
She dirties herself with the dirty salt-water; and
probably chills and tires herself by walking thither
and back, and staying in too long; and then flaunts on
the pier, bedizened in garments which, for monstrosity
of form and disharmony of colours, would have set that
Greek Nausicaa's teeth on edge, or those of any average
Hindoo woman now.   Or, even sadder still, she sits
on chairs and benches all the weary afternoon, her
head drooped on her chest, over some novel from the
" Library ; " and then returns to tea and shrimps, and
lodgings of which the fragrance is not unsuggestive,
sometimes not unproductive, of typhoid fever.   Ah, poor
Nausicaa of England !   That is a sad sight to some who
think about the present, and have read about the past.
It is not a sad sight to see your old father—tradesman,
or clerk, or what not—who has done good work in his day,
and hopes to do some more, sitting by your old mother,
who has done good work in her day—among the rest,
that heaviest work of all, the bringing you into the
world and keeping you in it till now—honest, kindly,
cheerful folk enough, and not inefficient in their own
calling; though an average Northumbrian, or Highlander, or Irish Easterling, beside carrying a brain of
five times the intellectual force, could drive five such men
over the cliff with his bare hands.   It is not a sad sight,

I say, to see them sitting about upon those seaside benches, looking out listlessly at the water, and the ships, and the sunlight, and enjoying, like so many flies upon a wall, the novel act of doing nothing. It is not the old for whom wise men are sad: but for you. Where is your vitality? Where is your "Lebensglückseligkeit," your enjoyment of superfluous life and power? Why can you not even dance and sing, till now and then, at night, perhaps, when you ought to be safe in bed, but when the weak brain, after receiving the day's nourishment, has roused itself a second time into a false excitement of gaslight pleasure? What there is left of it is all going into that foolish book, which the womanly element in you, still healthy and alive, delights in; because it places you in fancy in situations in which you will never stand, and inspires you with emotions, some of which, it may be, you had better never feel. Poor Nausicaa—old, some men think, before you have been ever young.

And now they are going to " develop " you; and let you have your share in "the higher education of women," by making you read more books, and do more sums, and pass examinations, and stoop over desks at night after stooping over some other employment all day; and to teach you Latin, and even Greek.

Well, we will gladly teach you Greek, if you learn thereby to read the history of Nausicaa of old, and what manner of maiden she was, and what was her education. You will admire her, doubtless. But do not let your admiration limit itself to drawing a meagre half-mediævalized design of her—as she never looked. Copy in your own person; and even if you do not descend as low—or rise as high—as washing the household clothes, at least learn to play at ball; and sing, in the open air and sunshine, not in theatres and concert-rooms by gaslight; and take decent care of your own health; and dress not like a "Parisienne"—nor, of course, like Nausicaa of old, for that is to ask too much :—but somewhat more like an average Highland lassie; and try to look like her, and be like her, of whom Wordsworth sang—

> "A mien and face
> In which full plainly I can trace
> Benignity, and home-bred sense,
> Ripening in perfect innocence.
> Here scattered, like a random seed,
> Remote from men, thou dost not need
> The embarrassed look of shy distress
> And maidenly shamefacedness.
> Thou wear'st upon thy forehead clear
> The freedom of a mountaineer.
> A face with gladness overspread,
> Soft smiles, by human kindness bred,
> And seemliness complete, that sways
> Thy courtesies, about thee plays.
> With no restraint, save such as springs
> From quick and eager visitings
> Of thoughts that lie beyond the reach
> Of thy few words of English speech.
> A bondage sweetly brooked, a strife
> That gives thy gestures grace and life."

Ah, yet unspoilt Nausicaa of the North; descendant of the dark tender-hearted Celtic girl, and the fair deep-hearted Scandinavian Viking, thank God for thy heather and fresh air, and the kine thou tendest, and the wool thou spinnest; and come not to seek thy fortune, child, in wicked London town; nor import, as they tell me thou art doing fast, the ugly fashions of that London town, clumsy copies of Parisian cockneydom, into thy Highland home; nor give up the healthful and graceful, free and modest dress of thy mother and thy mother's mother, to disfigure the little kirk on Sabbath days with crinoline and corset, high-heeled boots, and other women's hair.

It is proposed, just now, to assimilate the education of girls more and more to that of boys. If that means that girls are merely to learn more lessons, and to study what their brothers are taught, in addition to what their mothers were taught; then it is to be hoped, at least by physiologists and patriots, that the scheme will sink into that limbo whither, in a free and tolerably rational country, all imperfect and ill-considered schemes are sure to gravitate. But if the proposal be a bonâ fide one: then it must be borne in mind that in the public schools of England, and in all private schools, I presume, which take their tone from them, cricket and football are more or less compulsory, being considered integral parts of an Englishman's education;

and that they are likely to remain so, in spite of all
reclamations: because masters and boys alike know
that games do not, in the long run, interfere with a
boy's work; that the same boy will very often excel in
both; that the games keep him in health for his work;
and the spirit with which he takes to his games when
in the lower school, is a fair test of the spirit with which
he will take to his work when he rises into the higher
school; and that nothing is worse for a boy than to fall
into that loafing, tuck-shop-haunting set, who neither
play hard nor work hard, and are usually extravagant,
and often vicious. Moreover, they know well that
games conduce, not merely to physical, but to moral
health; that in the playing-field boys acquire virtues
which no books can give them; not merely daring and
endurance, but, better still, temper, self-restraint, fair-
ness, honour, unenvious approbation of another's success, and all that "give and take" of life which stand
a man in such good stead when he goes forth into the
world, and without which, indeed, his success is always
maimed and partial.

Now: if the promoters of higher education for women
will compel girls to any training analogous to our public
school games; if, for instance, they will insist on that
most natural and wholesome of all exercises, dancing,
in order to develop the lower half of the body; on
singing, to expand the lungs and regulate the breath;

and on some games—ball or what not—which will ensure that raised chest, and upright carriage, and general strength of the upper torso, without which full oxygenation of the blood, and therefore general health, is impossible; if they will sternly forbid tight stays, high heels, and all which interferes with free growth and free motion; if they will consider carefully all which has been written on the "half-time system" by Mr. Chadwick and others; and accept the certain physical law that, in order to renovate the brain day by day, the growing creature must have plenty of fresh air and play, and that the child who learns for four hours and plays for four hours, will learn more, and learn it more easily, than the child who learns for the whole eight hours; if, in short, they will teach girls not merely to understand the Greek tongue, but to copy somewhat of the Greek physical training, of that "music and gymnastic" which helped to make the cleverest race of the old world the ablest race likewise: then they will earn the gratitude of the patriot and the physiologist, by doing their best to stay the downward tendencies of the physique, and therefore ultimately of the morale, in the coming generation of English women.

I am sorry to say that, as yet, I hear of but one movement in this direction among the promoters of the

"higher education of women."* I trust that the subject
will be taken up methodically by those gifted ladies,
who have acquainted themselves, and are labouring to
acquaint other women, with the first principles of
health; and that they may avail to prevent the coming
generations, under the unwholesome stimulant of com-
petitive examinations, and so forth, from "developing" into so many Chinese——dwarfs—or idiots.

* Since this essay was written, I have been sincerely delighted to
find that my wishes had been anticipated at Girton College, near
Cambridge, and previously at Hitchin, whence the college was removed:
and that the wise ladies who superintend that establishment propose
also that most excellent institution—a swimming bath. A paper,
moreover, read before the London Association of Schoolmistresses in
1866, on "Physical Exercises and Recreation for Girls," deserves all
attention. May those who promote such things prosper as they
deserve.

THE AIR-MOTHERS.

" Die Natur ist die Bewegung."

WHO are these who follow us softly over the moor
in the autumn eve? Their wings brush and rustle in
the fir-boughs, and they whisper before us and behind,
as if they called gently to each other, like birds flocking
homeward to their nests.

The woodpecker on the pine-stems knows them, and
laughs aloud for joy as they pass. The rooks above
the pasture know them, and wheel round and tumble
in their play. The brown leaves on the oak trees
know them, and flutter faintly, and beckon as they
pass. And in the chattering of the dry leaves there is
a meaning, and a cry of weary things which long for
rest.

"Take us home, take us home, you soft air-mothers,
now our fathers the sunbeams are grown dull. Our
green summer beauty is all draggled, and our faces are
grown wan and wan; and the buds, the children whom
we nourished, thrust us off, ungrateful, from our seats.

Waft us down, you soft air-mothers, upon your wings to the quiet earth, that we may go to our home, as all things go, and become air and sunlight once again."

And the bold young fir-seeds know them, and rattle impatient in their cones. "Blow stronger, blow fiercer, slow air-mothers, and shake us from our prisons of dead wood, that we may fly and spin away north-eastward, each on his horny wing. Help us but to touch the moorland yonder, and we will take good care of ourselves henceforth; we will dive like arrows through the heather, and drive our sharp beaks into the soil, and rise again as green trees toward the sunlight, and spread out lusty boughs."

They never think, bold fools, of what is coming, to bring them low in the midst of their pride; of the reckless axe which will fell them, and the saw which will shape them into logs; and the trains which will roar and rattle over them, as they lie buried in the gravel of the way, till they are ground and rotted into powder, and dug up and flung upon the fire, that they too may return home, like all things, and become air and sunlight once again.

And the air-mothers hear their prayers, and do their bidding: but faintly; for they themselves are tired and sad.

Tired and sad are the air-mothers, and their garments rent and wan. Look at them as they stream

over the black forest, before the dim south-western
sun; long lines and wreaths of melancholy grey, stained
with dull yellow or dead dun. They have come far
across the seas, and done many a wild deed upon their
way; and now that they have reached the land, like
shipwrecked sailors, they will lie down and weep till
they can weep no more.

Ah, how different were those soft air-mothers when,
invisible to mortal eyes, they started on their long sky-
journey, five thousand miles across the sea! Out of
the blazing caldron which lies between the two New
Worlds, they leapt up when the great sun called them,
in whirls and spouts of clear hot steam; and rushed
of their own passion to the northward, while the
whirling earth-ball whirled them east. So north-
eastward they rushed aloft, across the gay West
Indian isles, leaving below the glitter of the flying-
fish, and the sidelong eyes of cruel sharks; above the
cane-fields and the plaintain-gardens, and the cocoa-
groves which fringe the shores; above the rocks which
throbbed with earthquakes, and the peaks of old vol-
canoes, cinder-strewn; while, far beneath, the ghosts
of their dead sisters hurried home upon the north-east
breeze.

Wild deeds they did as they rushed onward, and
struggled and fought among themselves, up and down,
and round and backward, in the fury of their blind hot

youth. They heeded not the tree as they snapped it, nor the ship as they whelmed it in the waves; nor the cry of the sinking sailor, nor the need of his little ones on shore; hasty and selfish even as children, and, like children, tamed by their own rage. For they tired themselves by struggling with each other, and by tearing the heavy water into waves; and their wings grew clogged with sea-spray, and soaked more and more with steam. But at last the sea grew cold beneath them, and their clear steam shrank to mist; and they saw themselves and each other wrapped in dull rain-laden clouds. They then drew their white cloud-garments round them, and veiled themselves for very shame; and said, "We have been wild and wayward: and, alas! our pure bright youth is gone. But we will do one good deed yet ere we die, and so we shall not have lived in vain. We will glide onward to the land, and weep there; and refresh all things with soft warm rain; and make the grass grow, the buds burst; quench the thirst of man and beast, and wash the soiled world clean."

So they are wandering past us, the air-mothers, to weep the leaves into their graves; to weep the seeds into their seed-beds, and weep the soil into the plains; to get the rich earth ready for the winter, and then creep northward to the ice-world, and there die.

Weary, and still more weary, slowly, and more slowly

still, they will journey on far northward, across fast-chilling seas. For a doom is laid upon them, never to be still again, till they rest at the North Pole itself, the still axle of the spinning world; and sink in death around it, and become white snow-clad ghosts.

But will they live again, those chilled air-mothers? Yes, they must live again. For all things move for ever; and not even ghosts can rest. So the corpses of their sisters, piling on them from above, press them outward, press them southward toward the sun once more; across the floes and round the icebergs, weeping tears of snow and sleet, while men hate their wild harsh voices, and shrink before their bitter breath. They know not that the cold bleak snow-storms, as they hurtle from the black north-east, bear back the ghosts of the soft air-mothers, as penitents, to their father, the great sun.

But as they fly southwards, warm life thrills them, and they drop their loads of sleet and snow; and meet their young live sisters from the south, and greet them with flash and thunder-peal. And, please God, before many weeks are over, as we run Westward Ho, we shall overtake the ghosts of these air-mothers, hurrying back toward their father, the great sun. Fresh and bright under the fresh bright heaven, they will race with us toward our home, to gain new heat, new life, new power, and set forth about their work

once more.   Men call them the south-west wind, those
air-mothers ; and their ghosts the north-east trade ; and
value them, and rightly, because they bear the traders
out and home across the sea.   But wise men, and little
children, should look on them with more seeing eyes ;
and say, " May not these winds be living creatures ?
They, too, are thoughts of God, to whom all live."

For is not our life like their life ?   Do we not come
and go as they ?   Out of God's boundless bosom, the
fount of life, we came ; through selfish, stormy youth
and contrite tears—just not too late ; through manhood not altogether useless ; through slow and chill
old age, we return from Whence we came ; to the
Bosom of God once more—to go forth again, it may
be, with fresh knowledge, and fresh powers, to nobler
work.   Amen.

Such was the prophecy which I learnt, or seemed to
learn, from the south-western wind off the Atlantic, on
a certain delectable evening.   And it was fulfilled at
night, as far as the gentle air-mothers could fulfil it,
for foolish man.

> " There was a roaring in the woods all night ;
> The rain came heavily and fell in floods ;
> But now the sun is rising calm and bright,
> The birds are singing in the distant woods ;
> Over his own sweet voice the stock-dove broods,
> The jay makes answer as the magpie chatters,
> And all the air is filled with pleasant noise of waters."

But was I a gloomy and distempered man, if, upon such a morn as that, I stood on the little bridge across a certain brook, and watched the water run, with something of a sigh? Or if, when the schoolboy beside me lamented that the floods would surely be out, and his day's fishing spoiled, I said to him—"Ah, my boy, that is a little matter. Look at what you are seeing now, and understand what barbarism and waste mean. Look at all that beautiful water which God has sent us hither off the Atlantic, without trouble or expense to us. Thousands, and tens of thousands, of gallons will run under this bridge to-day; and what shall we do with it? Nothing. And yet: think only of the mills which that water would have turned. Think how it might have kept up health and cleanliness in poor creatures packed away in the back streets of the near-est town, or even in London itself. Think even how country folks, in many parts of England, in three months' time, may be crying out for rain, and afraid of short crops, and fever, and scarlatina, and cattle-plague, for want of the very water which we are now letting run back, wasted, into the sea from whence it came. And yet we call ourselves a civilised people."

It is not wise, I know, to preach to boys. And yet, sometimes, a man must speak his heart; even, like Midas' slave, to the reeds by the river side. And I had so often, fishing up and down full many a stream, whispered my story to those same river-reeds; and told them that my Lord the Sovereign Demos had, like old Midas, asses' ears in spite of all his gold, that I thought I might for once tell it the boy likewise, in hope that he might help his generation to mend that which my own generation does not seem like to mend.

I might have said more to him: but did not. For it is not well to destroy too early the child's illusion, that people must be wise because they are grown up, and have votes, and rule—or think they rule—the world. The child will find out how true that is soon enough for himself. If the truth be forced on him by the hot words of those with whom he lives, it is apt to breed in him that contempt, stormful and therefore barren, which makes revolutions; and not that pity, calm and therefore helpful, which makes reforms.

So I might have said to him, but did not——

And then men pray for rain:

My boy, did you ever hear the old Eastern legend about the Gipsies? How they were such good musicians, that some great Indian Sultan sent for the whole tribe, and planted them near his palace, and gave them land, and ploughs to break it up, and seed to sow it, that they might dwell there, and play and sing to him.

But when the winter arrived, the Gipsies all came to the Sultan, and cried that they were starving. "But what have you done with the seed-corn which I gave you?" "O Light of the Age, we ate it in the summer." "And what have you done with the ploughs which I gave you?" "O Glory of the Universe, we burnt them to bake the corn withal."

Then said that great Sultan—"Like the butterflies you have lived; and like the butterflies you shall wander." So he drove them out. And that is how the Gipsies came hither from the East.

Now suppose that the Sultan of all Sultans, who sends the rain, should make a like answer to us foolish human beings, when we prayed for rain: "But what have you done with the rain which I gave you six months since?" "We have let it run into the sea." "Then, ere you ask for more rain, make places wherein you can keep it when you have it." "But that would be, in most cases, too expensive. We can employ our capital more profitably in other directions."

It is not for me to say what answer might be made to such an excuse. I think a child's still unsophisticated sense of right and wrong would soon supply one; and probably one—considering the complexity, and difficulty, and novelty, of the whole question— somewhat too harsh; as children's judgments are wont to be.

But would it not be well if our children, without being taught to blame any one for what is past, were taught something about what ought to be done now, what must be done soon, with the rainfall of these islands; and about other and kindred health-questions, on the solution of which depends, and will depend more and more, the life of millions? One would have thought that those public schools and colleges which desire to monopolise the education of the owners of the soil; of the great employers of labour; of the clergy; and of all, indeed, who ought to be acquainted with the duties of property, the conditions of public health, and, in a word, with the general laws of what is now called Social Science—one would have thought, I say, that these public schools and colleges would have taught their scholars somewhat at least about such matters, that they might go forth into life with at least some rough notions of the causes which make people healthy or unhealthy, rich or poor, comfortable or wretched, useful or dangerous to the State. But as long as our great educational institutions, safe, or fancying themselves safe, in some enchanted castle, shut out by ancient magic from the living world, put a premium on Latin and Greek verses: a wise father will, during the holidays, talk now and then, I hope, somewhat after this fashion :—

You must understand, my boy, that all the water

in the country comes out of the sky, and from nowhere else; and that, therefore, to save and store the water when it falls is a question of life and death to crops, and man, and beast; for with or without water is life or death. If I took, for instance, the water from the moors above and turned it over yonder field, I could double, and more than double, the crops in that field, henceforth.

Then why do I not do it?

Only because the field lies higher than the house; and if—now here is one thing which you and every civilised man should know—if you have water-meadows, or any "irrigated" land, as it is called, above a house, or even on a level with it, it is certain to breed not merely cold and damp, but fever or ague. Our forefathers did not understand this; and they built their houses, as this is built, in the lowest places they could find: sometimes because they wished to be near ponds, from whence they could get fish in Lent; but more often, I think, because they wanted to be sheltered from the wind. They had no glass, as we have, in their windows; or, at least, only latticed casements, which let in the wind and cold; and they shrank from high and exposed, and therefore really healthy, spots. But now that we have good glass, and sash windows, and doors that will shut tight, we can build warm houses where we like. And if you ever have to do with the

building of cottages, remember that it is your duty to
the people who will live in them, and therefore to the
State, to see that they stand high and dry, where no water
can drain down into their foundations, and where fog,
and the poisonous gases which are given out by rotting
vegetables, cannot drain down either. You will learn
more about all that when you learn, as every civilised
lad should in these days, something about chemistry,
and the laws of fluids and gases. But you know
already that flowers are cut off by frost in the low
grounds sooner than in the high; and that the fog at
night always lies along the brooks; and that the sour
moor-smell which warns us to shut our windows at
sunset, comes down from the hill, and not up from the
valley. Now all these things are caused by one and
the same law; that cold air is heavier than warm;
and, therefore, like so much water, must run down-
hill.

But what about the rainfall?

Well, I have wandered a little from the rainfall:
though not as far as you fancy; for fever and ague and
rheumatism usually mean—rain in the wrong place. But
if you knew how much illness, and torturing pain, and
death, and sorrow arise, even to this very day, from
ignorance of these simple laws, then you would bear
them carefully in mind, and wish to know more about
them. But now for water being life to the beasts.

Do you remember—though you are hardly old enough —the cattle-plague? How the beasts died, or had to be killed and buried, by tens of thousands; and how misery and ruin fell on hundreds of honest men and women over many of the richest counties of England : but how we in this vale had no cattle-plague ; and how there was none—as far as I recollect—in the uplands of Devon and Cornwall, nor of Wales, nor of the Scotch Highlands ? Now, do you know why that was ? Simply because we here, like those other up-landers, are in such a country as Palestine was before the foolish Jews cut down all their timber, and so destroyed their own rainfall—a "land of brooks of water, of fountains and depths that spring out of valleys and hills." There is hardly a field here that has not, thank God, its running brook, or its sweet spring, from which our cattle were drinking their health and life, while in the clay-lands of Cheshire, and in the Cambridgeshire fens—which were drained utterly dry —the poor things drank no water, too often, save that of the very same putrid ponds in which they had been standing all day long, to cool themselves, and to keep off the flies. I do not say, of course, that bad water caused the cattle-plague. It came by infection from the East of Europe. But I say that bad water made the cattle ready to take it, and made it spread over the country; and when you are old enough I will give you

plenty of proof—some from the herds of your own
kinsmen—that what I say is true.

And as for pure water being life to human beings :
why have we never fever here, and scarcely ever diseases
like fever—zymotics, as the doctors call them ?   Or, if a
case comes into our parish from outside, why does the
fever never spread ?   For the very same reason that we
had no cattle-plague.   Because we have more pure
water close to every cottage than we need.   And this I
tell you : that the only two outbreaks of deadly disease
which we have had here for thirty years, were both of
them, as far as I could see, to be traced to filthy water
having got into the poor folk's wells.   Water, you
must remember, just as it is life when pure, is death
when foul.   For it can carry, unseen to the eye, and
even when it looks clear and sparkling, and tastes soft
and sweet, poisons which have perhaps killed more
human beings than ever were killed in battle.   You
have read, perhaps, how the Athenians, when they were
dying of the plague, accused the Lacedæmonians outside the walls of poisoning their wells; or how, in some
of the pestilences of the middle ages, the common
people used to accuse the poor harmless Jews of poisoning the wells, and set upon them and murdered them
horribly.   They were right, I do not doubt, in their
notion that the well-water was giving them the pestilence : but they had not sense to see that they were

poisoning the wells themselves by their dirt and carelessness; or, in the case of poor besieged Athens, probably by mere overcrowding, which has cost many a
life ere now, and will cost more. And I am sorry to
tell you, my little man, that even now too many people
have no more sense than they had, and die in consequence. If you could see a battle-field, and men shot
down, writhing and dying in hundreds by shell and
bullet, would not that seem to you a horrid sight?
Then—I do not wish to make you sad too early, but
this is a fact that every one should know—that more
people, and not strong men only, but women and little
children too, are killed and wounded in Great Britain
every year by bad water and want of water together,
than were killed and wounded in any battle which has
been fought since you were born. Medical men know
this well. And when you are older, you may see it for
yourself in the Registrar-General's reports, blue-books,
pamphlets, and so on, without end.

But why do not people stop such a horrible loss of
life?

Well, my dear boy, the true causes of it have only
been known for the last thirty or forty years; and we
English are, as good King Alfred found us to his sorrow
a thousand years ago, very slow to move, even when we
see a thing ought to be done. Let us hope that in this
matter—we have been so in most matters as yet—we

shall be like the tortoise in the fable, and not the hare ;
and by moving slowly, but surely, win the race at last.
But now think for yourself : and see what you would do
to save these people from being poisoned by bad water.
Remember that the plain question is this—The rain-
water comes down from heaven as water, and nothing
but water. Rain-water is the only pure water, after
all. How would you save that for the poor people who
have none ? There ; run away and hunt rabbits on the
moor : but look, meanwhile, how you would save some
of this beautiful and precious water which is roaring
away into the sea.

*   *   *   *   *

Well ? What would you do ? Make ponds, you
say, like the old monks' ponds, now all broken down.
Dam all the glens across their mouths, and turn them
into reservoirs.

"Out of the mouths of babes and sucklings "——
Well, that will have to be done. That is being done
more and more, more or less well. The good people of
Glasgow did it first, I think ; and now the good people
of Manchester, and of other northern towns, have done
it, and have saved many a human life thereby already.
But it must be done, some day, all over England and
Wales, and great part of Scotland. For the mountain
tops and moors, my boy, by a beautiful law of nature,
compensate for their own poverty by yielding a wealth

which the rich lowlands cannot yield. You do not understand? Then see. Yon moor above can grow neither corn nor grass. But one thing it can grow, and does grow, without which we should have no corn nor grass, and that is—water. Not only does far more rain fall up there than falls here down below, but even in drought the high moors condense the moisture into dew, and so yield some water, even when the lowlands are burnt up with drought. The reason of that you must learn hereafter. That it is so, you should know yourself. For on the high chalk downs, you know, where farmers make a sheep-pond, they never, if they are wise, make it in a valley or on a hillside, but on the bleakest top of the very highest down; and there, if they can once get it filled with snow and rain in winter, the blessed dews of night will keep some water in it all the summer through, while the ponds below are utterly dried up. And even so it is, as I know, with this very moor. Corn and grass it will not grow, because there is too little " staple," that is, soluble minerals, in the sandy soil. But how much water it might grow, you may judge roughly for yourself, by remembering how many brooks like this are running off it now to carry mere dirt into the river, and then into the sea.

But why should we not make dams at once; and save the water?

Because we cannot afford it. No one would buy

the water when we had stored it. The rich in town and country will always take care—and quite right they are—to have water enough for themselves, and for their servants too, whatever it may cost them. But the poorer people are—and therefore usually, alas! the more ignorant—the less water they get; and the less they care to have water; and the less they are inclined to pay for it; and the more, I am sorry to say, they waste what little they do get; and I am still more sorry to say, spoil, and even steal and sell—in London at least—the stop-cocks and lead-pipes which bring the water into their houses. So that keeping a water-shop is a very troublesome and uncertain business; and one which is not likely to pay us or any one round here.

But why not let some company manage it, as they manage railways, and gas, and other things?

Ah—you have been overhearing a good deal about companies of late, I see. But this I will tell you; that when you grow up, and have a vote and influence, it will be your duty, if you intend to be a good citizen, not only not to put the water-supply of England into the hands of fresh companies, but to help to take out of their hands what water-supply they manage already, especially in London; and likewise the gas-supply; and the railroads; and everything else, in a word, which everybody uses, and must use. For you must understand

—at least as soon as you can—that though the men who make up companies are no worse than other men, and some of them, as you ought to know, very good men; yet what they have to look to is their profits; and the less water they supply, and the worse it is, the more profit they make. For most water, I am sorry to say, is fouled before the water companies can get to it, as this water which runs past us will be, and as the Thames water above London is. Therefore it has to be cleansed, or partly cleansed, at a very great expense. So water companies have to be inspected—in plain English, watched—at a very heavy expense to the nation by government officers ; and compelled to do their best, and take their utmost care. And so it has come to pass that the London water is not now nearly as bad as some of it was thirty years ago, when it was no more fit to drink than that in the cattle-yard tank. But still we must have more water, and better, in London; for it is growing year by year. There are more than three millions of people already in what we call London ; and ere you are an old man there may be between four and five millions. Now to supply all these people with water is a duty which we must not leave to any private companies. It must be done by a public authority, as is fit and proper in a free self-governing country. In this matter, as in all others, we will try to do what the Royal Commission told us four years

ago we ought to do. I hope that you will see, though
I may not, the day when what we call London, but
which is really, nine-tenths of it, only a great nest of
separate villages huddled together, will be divided into
three great self-governing cities, London, Westminster,
and Southwark; each with its own corporation, like
that of the venerable and well-governed City of London; each managing its own water-supply, gas-supply,
and sewage, and other matters besides; and managing
them, like Dublin, Glasgow, Manchester, Liverpool, and
other great northern towns, far more cheaply and far
better than any companies can do it for them.

But where shall we get water enough for all these
millions of people? There are no mountains near
London. But we might give them the water off our
moors.

No, no, my boy.

> "He that will not when he may,
> When he will, he shall have nay."

Some fifteen years ago the Londoners might have had
water from us; and I was one of those who did my
best to get it for them: but the water companies did
not chose to take it; and now this part of England
is growing so populous and so valuable that it wants
all its little rainfall for itself. So there is another leaf
torn out of the Sibylline books for the poor old water
companies. You do not understand: you will some

day. But you may comfort yourself about London. For it happens to be, I think, the luckiest city in the world; and if it had not been, we should have had pestilence on pestilence in it, as terrible as the great plague of Charles II.'s time. The old Britons, without knowing in the least what they were doing, settled old London city in the very centre of the most wonderful natural reservoir in this island, or perhaps in all Europe; which reaches from Kent into Wiltshire, and round again into Suffolk; and that is, the dear old chalk downs.

Why, they are always dry.

Yes. But the turf on them never burns up, and the streams which flow through them never run dry, and seldom or never flood either. Do you not know, from Winchester, that that is true? Then where is all the rain and snow gone, which falls on them year by year, but into the chalk itself, and into the greensands, too, below the chalk? There it is, soaked up as by a sponge, in quantity incalculable; enough, some think, to supply London, let it grow as huge as it may. I wish I too were sure of that. But the Commission has shown itself so wise and fair, and brave likewise—too brave, I am sorry to say, for some who might have supported them—that it is not for me to gainsay their opinion.

But if there was not water enough in the chalk, are

not the Londoners rich enough to bring it from any distance?

My boy, in this also we will agree with the Commission—that we ought not to rob Peter to pay Paul, and take water to a distance which other people close at hand may want. Look at the map of England and southern Scotland; and see for yourself what is just, according to geography and nature. There are four mountain-ranges; four great water-fields. First, the hills of the Border. Their rainfall ought to be stored for the Lothians and the extreme north of England. Then the Yorkshire and Derbyshire Hills—the central chine of England. Their rainfall is being stored already, to the honour of the shrewd northern men, for the manufacturing counties east and west of the hills. Then come the lake mountains—the finest water-field of all, because more rain by far falls there than in any place in England. But they will be wanted to supply Lancashire, and some day Liverpool itself; for Liverpool is now using rain which belongs more justly to other towns; and besides, there are plenty of counties and towns, down into Cheshire, which would be glad of what water Lancashire does not want. And last come the Snowdon mountains, a noble water-field, which I know well; for an old dream of mine has been, that ere I died I should see all the rain of the Carnedds, and the Glyders, and Siabod, and Snowdon itself, car-

ried across the Conway river to feed the mining districts
of North Wales, where the streams are now all foul with
oil and lead; and then on into the western coal and
iron fields, to Wolverhampton and Birmingham itself:
and if I were the engineer who got that done, I should
be happier—prouder I dare not say—than if I had
painted nobler pictures than Raffaelle, or written nobler
plays than Shakespeare. I say that, boy, in most de-
liberate earnest. But meanwhile, do you not see that
in districts where coal and iron may be found, and
fresh manufactures may spring up any day in any
place, each district has a right to claim the nearest
rainfall for itself? And now, when we have got the
water into its proper place, let us see what we shall do
with it.

But why do you say we? Can you and I do all
this?

My boy, are not you and I free citizens; part of
the people, the Commons—as the good old word runs—
of this country? And are we not—or ought we not to
be in time—beside that, educated men? By the people, remember, I mean, not only the hand-working man
who has just got a vote; I mean the clergy of all de-
nominations; and the gentlemen of the press; and last,
but not least, the scientific men. If those four classes
together were to tell every government—"Free water
we will have, and as much as we reasonably choose;"

and tell every candidate for the House of Commons,—
" Unless you promise to get us as much free water as
we reasonably choose, we will not return you to Parliament :" then, I think, we four should put such a "pressure " on government as no water companies, or other
vested interests, could long resist.   And if any of those
four classes should hang back, and waste their time and
influence over matters far less important and less press-
ing, the other three must laugh at them, and more
than laugh at them ; and ask them—" Why have you
education, why have you influence, why have you votes,
why are you freemen and not slaves, if not to preserve
the comfort, the decency, the health, the lives of men,
women, and children—most of those latter your own
wives and your own children ? "

But what shall we do with the water ?

Well, after all, that is a more practical matter than
speculations grounded on the supposition that all
classes will do their duty.   But the first thing we will
do will be to give to the very poorest houses a constant
supply, at high pressure ; so that everybody may take
as much water as he likes, instead of having to keep
the water in little cisterns, where it gets foul and
putrid only too often.

But will they not waste it then ?

So far from it, wherever the water has been laid on at
high pressure, the waste, which is terrible now—some

say that in London one-third of the water is wasted—
begins to lessen; and both water and expense are saved.
If you will only think, you will see one reason why. If
a woman leaves a high-pressure tap running, she will
flood her place and her neighbour's too. She will be
like the magician's servant, who called up the demon
to draw water for him; and so he did: but when he
had begun he would not stop, and if the magician had
not come home, man and house would have been washed
away.

But if it saves money, why do not the water companies do it?

Because—and really here there are many excuses for
the poor old water companies, when so many of them
swerve and gib at the very mention of constant water-
supply, like a poor horse set to draw a load which he
feels is too heavy for him—because, to keep everything
in order among dirty, careless, and often drunken
people, there must be officers with lawful authority—
water-policemen we will call them—who can enter
people's houses when they will, and if they find anything wrong with the water, set it to rights with a
high hand, and even summon the people who have set
it wrong. And that is a power which, in a free country,
must never be given to the servants of any private
company, but only to the officers of a corporation or of
the government.

I

And what shall we do with the rest of the water?

Well, we shall have, I believe, so much to spare that we may at least do this—In each district of each city, and the centre of each town, we may build public baths and lavatories, where poor men and women may get their warm baths when they will; for now they usually never bathe at all, because they will not—and ought not, if they be hard-worked folk—bathe in cold water during nine months of the year. And there they shall wash their clothes, and dry them by steam; instead of washing them as now, at home, either under back sheds, where they catch cold and rheumatism, or too often, alas! in their own living rooms, in an atmosphere of foul vapour, which drives the father to the public-house and the children into the streets; and which not only prevents the clothes from being thoroughly dried again, but is, my dear boy, as you will know when you are older, a very hot-bed of disease. And they shall have other comforts, and even luxuries, these public lavatories; and be made, in time, graceful and refining, as well as merely useful. Nay, we will even, I think, have in front of each of them a real fountain; not like the drinking-fountains—though they are great and needful boons—which you see here and there about the streets, with a tiny dribble of water to a great deal of expensive stone: but real fountains, which shall leap, and sparkle, and plash, and gurgle;

and fill the place with life, and light, and coolness; and sing in the people's ears the sweetest of all earthly songs —save the song of a mother over her child—the song of " The Laughing Water."

But will not that be a waste?

Yes, my boy. And for that very reason, I think we, the people, will have our fountains; if it be but to make our governments, and corporations, and all public bodies and officers, remember that they all— save Her Majesty the Queen—are our servants; and not we theirs; and that we choose to have water, not only to wash with, but to play with, if we like. And I believe—for the world, as you will find, is full not only of just but of generous souls—that if the water-supply were set really right, there would be found, in many a city, many a generous man who, over and above his compulsory water-rate, would give his poor fellow-townsmen such a real fountain as those which ennoble the great square at Carcasonne and the great square at Nismes; to be " a thing of beauty and a joy for ever."

And now, if you want to go back to your Latin and Greek, you shall translate for me into Latin—I do not expect you to do it into Greek, though it would turn very well into Greek, for the Greeks knew all about the matter long before the Romans—what follows here; and you shall verify the facts and the names,

&c., in it from your dictionaries of antiquity and biography, that you may remember all the better what it says. And by that time, I think, you will have learnt something more useful to yourself, and, I hope, to your country hereafter, than if you had learnt to patch together the neatest Greek and Latin verses which have appeared since the days of Mr. Canning.

    *   *   *   *   *

I have often amused myself, by fancying one question which an old Roman emperor would ask, were he to rise from his grave and visit the sights of London under the guidance of some minister of state. The august shade would, doubtless, admire our railroads and bridges, our cathedrals and our public parks, and much more of which we need not be ashamed. But after a while, I think, he would look round, whether in London or in most of our great cities, inquiringly and in vain, for one class of buildings, which in his empire were wont to be almost as conspicuous and as splendid, because, in public opinion, almost as necessary, as the basilicas and temples—"And where," he would ask, "are your public baths?" And if the minister of state who was his guide should answer—"O great Cæsar, I really do not know. I believe there are some somewhere at the back of that ugly building which we call the National Gallery; and I think there have been some meetings lately in the East End, and an amateur concert at the Albert Hall, for restoring, by private subscriptions, some baths and wash-houses in Bethnal Green, which had fallen to decay. And there may be two or three more about the metropolis; for parish vestries have powers by Act of Parliament to establish such places, if they think fit, and choose to pay for them out of the rates: "—Then, I think, the august shade might well make answer—"We used to call you, in old Rome, northern barbarians. It seems that you have not lost all your barbarian habits. Are you aware that, in every city in the Roman empire, there were, as a matter of course, public baths open, not only to the poorest freeman, but to the slave, usually for the payment of the smallest current coin, and often gratuitously? Are you aware that in Rome itself, millionaire after millionaire, emperor after emperor, from Menenius Agrippa and Nero down to Diocletian and Constantine, built baths, and yet more baths; and connected with them gymnasia for exercise, lecture-rooms, libraries, and porticos, wherein the people might have shade and shelter, and rest?—I remark, by-the-by, that I have not seen in all your London a single covered place in which the people may take shelter during a shower—Are you aware that these baths were of the most magnificent architecture, decorated with marbles, paintings, sculptures, fountains, what not? And yet I had heard, in Hades down below, that you prided yourselves here on the study of the learned languages; and, indeed, taught little but Greek and Latin at your public schools?"

Then, if the minister should make reply—"Oh yes, we know all this. Even since the revival of letters in the end of the fifteenth century a whole literature has been written—a great deal of it, I fear, by pedants who seldom washed even their hands and faces—about your Greek and Roman baths. We visit their colossal ruins in Italy and elsewhere with awe and admiration; and the discovery of a new Roman bath in any old city of our isles sets all our antiquaries buzzing with interest."

"Then why," the shade might ask, "do you not copy an example which you so much admire? Surely England must be much in want, either of water, or of fuel to heat it with?"

"On the contrary, our rainfall is almost too great; our soil so damp that we have had to invent a whole art of subsoil drainage unknown to you; while, as for fuel, our coal-mines make us the great fuel-exporting people of the world."

What a quiet sneer might curl the lip of a Constantine as he replied—"Not in vain, as I said, did we call you, some fifteen hundred years ago, the barbarians of the north. But tell me, good barbarian, whom I know to be both brave and wise—for the fame of your young British empire has reached us even in the realms below, and we recognise in you, with all respect, a people more like us Romans than any which has appeared on earth for many centuries—how is it you have forgotten that sacred duty of keeping the people clean, which you surely at one time learnt from us? When your ancestors entered our armies, and rose, some of them, to be great generals, and even emperors, like those two Teuton peasants, Justin and Justinian, who, long after my days, reigned in my own Constantinople: then, at least, you saw baths, and used them; and felt, after the bath, that you were civilised men, and not 'sordidi ac fœtentes,' as we used to call you when fresh out of your bullock-waggons and cattle-pens. How is it that you have forgotten that lesson?"

The minister, I fear, would have to answer that our ancestors were barbarous enough, not only to destroy the Roman cities, and temples, and basilicas, and statues, but the Roman baths likewise ; and then retired, each man to his own freehold in the country, to live a life not much more cleanly or more graceful than that of the swine which were his favourite food. But he would have a right to plead, as an excuse, that not only in England, but throughout the whole of the conquered Latin empire, the Latin priesthood, who, in some respects, were—to their honour—the representatives of Roman civilisation and the protectors of its remnants,

were the determined enemies of its cleanliness; that
they looked on personal dirt—like the old hermits of
the Thebaid—as a sign of sanctity; and discouraged—
as they are said to do still in some of the Romance
countries of Europe—the use of the bath, as not only
luxurious, but also indecent.

At which answer, it seems to me, another sneer
might curl the lip of the august shade, as he said to
himself—"This, at least, I did not expect, when I
made Christianity the state religion of my empire.
But you, good barbarian, look clean enough. You do
not look on dirt as a sign of sanctity?"

"On the contrary, sire, the upper classes of our
empire boast of being the cleanliest—perhaps the only
perfectly cleanly—people in the world: except, of
course, the savages of the South Seas. And dirt is so far
from being a thing which we admire, that our scientific
men—than whom the world has never seen wiser—have
proved to us, for a whole generation past, that dirt is
the fertile cause of disease and drunkenness, misery
and recklessness."

"And, therefore," replies the shade, ere he disap-
pears, "of discontent and revolution: followed by a
tyranny endured, as in Rome and many another place,
by men once free; because tyranny will at least do for
them what they are too lazy, and cowardly, and greedy
to do for themselves. Farewell, and prosper; as you

seem likely to prosper, on the whole. But if you wish me to consider you a civilised nation : let me hear that you have brought a great river from the depths of the earth, be they a thousand fathoms deep, or from your nearest mountains, be they five hundred miles away; and have washed out London's dirt—and your own shame. Till then, abstain from judging too harshly a Constantine, or even a Caracalla; for they, whatever were their sins, built baths, and kept their people clean. But do your gymnasia—your schools and universities, teach your youth nought about all this?"

THRIFT.

A LECTURE DELIVERED AT WINCHESTER, MARCH 17, 1869.

———◦◦◦———

LADIES,—I have chosen for the title of this lecture a practical and prosaic word, because I intend the lecture itself to be as practical and prosaic as I can make it, without becoming altogether dull.

The question of the better or worse education of women is one far too important for vague sentiment, wild aspirations, or Utopian dreams.

It is a practical question, on which depends not merely money or comfort, but too often health and life, as the consequences of a good education, or disease and death—I know too well of what I speak—as the consequences of a bad one.

I beg you, therefore, to put out of your minds at the outset any fancy that I wish for a social revolution in the position of women; or that I wish to see them educated by exactly the same methods, and in exactly the same subjects, as men. British lads, on an average, are far too ill-taught still, in spite of all recent improvements, for me to wish that British girls should be taught in the same way.

Moveover, whatever defects there may have been—and defects there must be in all things human—in the past education of British women, it has been most certainly a splendid moral success. It has made, by the grace of God, British women the best wives, mothers, daughters, aunts, sisters, that the world, as far as I can discover, has yet seen.

Let those who will sneer at the women of England. We who have to do the work and to fight the battle of life know the inspiration which we derive from their virtue, their counsel, their tenderness, and—but too often—from their compassion and their forgiveness. There is, I doubt not, still left in England many a man with chivalry and patriotism enough to challenge the world to show so perfect a specimen of humanity as a cultivated British woman.

But just because a cultivated British woman is so perfect a personage; therefore I wish to see all British women cultivated. Because the womanhood of England is so precious a treasure; I wish to see none of it wasted. It is an invaluable capital, or material, out of which the greatest possible profit to the nation must be made. And that can only be done by thrift; and that, again, can only be attained by knowledge.

Consider that word thrift. If you will look at Dr. Johnson's Dictionary, or if you know your Shakespeare, you will see that thrift signified originally profits, gain, riches gotten—in a word, the marks of a man's thriving.

How, then, did the word thrift get to mean parsimony, frugality, the opposite of waste? Just in the same way as economy—which first, of course, meant the management of a household—got to mean also the opposite of waste.

It was found that in commerce, in husbandry, in any process, in fact, men throve in proportion as they saved their capital, their material, their force.

Now this is a great law which runs through life; one of those laws of nature—call them, rather, laws of God—which apply not merely to political economy, to commerce, and to mechanics; but to physiology, to society; to the intellect, to the heart, of every person in this room.

The secret of thriving is thrift; saving of force; to get as much work as possible done with the least expenditure of power, the least jar and obstruction, the least wear and tear.

And the secret of thrift is knowledge. In proportion as you know the laws and nature of a subject, you will be able to work at it easily, surely, rapidly, successfully; instead of wasting your money or your energies in mistaken schemes, irregular efforts, which end in disappointment and exhaustion.

The secret of thrift, I say, is knowledge. The more you know, the more you can save yourself and that which belongs to you; and can do more work with less effort.

A knowledge of the laws of commercial credit, we all know, saves capital, enabling a less capital to do the work of a greater. Knowledge of the electric telegraph saves time; knowledge of writing saves human speech and locomotion; knowledge of domestic economy saves income; knowledge of sanitary laws saves health and life; knowledge of the laws of the intellect saves wear and tear of brain; and knowledge of the laws of the spirit—what does it not save?

A well-educated moral sense, a well-regulated character, saves from idleness and ennui, alternating with sentimentality and excitement, those tenderer emotions, those deeper passions, those nobler aspirations of humanity, which are the heritage of the woman far more than of the man; and which are potent in her, for evil or for good, in proportion as they are left to run wild and undisciplined, or are trained and developed into graceful, harmonious, self-restraining strength, beautiful in themselves, and a blessing to all who come under their influence.

What, therefore, I recommend to ladies in this lecture is thrift: thrift of themselves and of their own powers: and knowledge as the parent of thrift.

And because it is well to begin with the lower applications of thrift, and to work up to the higher, I am much pleased to hear that the first course of the proposed lectures to women in this place will be one on domestic economy.

I presume that the learned gentleman who will deliver these lectures will be the last to mean by that term the mere saving of money: that he will tell you, as—being a German—he will have good reason to know, that the young lady who learns thrift in domestic economy is also learning thrift of the very highest faculties of her immortal spirit. He will tell you, I doubt not—for he must know—how you may see in Germany young ladies living in what we more luxurious British would consider something like poverty; cooking, waiting at table, and performing many a household office which would be here considered menial; and yet finding time for a cultivation of the intellect, which is, unfortunately, too rare in Great Britain.

The truth is, that we British are too wealthy. We make money, if not too rapidly for the good of the nation at large, yet too rapidly, I fear, for the good of the daughters of those who make it. Their temptation—I do not, of course, say they all yield to it—but their temptation is, to waste of the very simplest—I had almost said, if I may be pardoned the expression, of the most barbaric—kind; to an oriental waste of money, and waste of time; to a fondness for mere finery, pardonable enough, but still a waste; and to the mistaken fancy that it is the mark of a lady to sit idle and let servants do everything for her.

Such women may well take a lesson by contrast from the pure and noble, useful and cultivated thrift of an average German young lady—for ladies these German women are, in every possible sense of the word.

But it is not of this sort of waste of which I wish to speak to-day. I only mention the matter in passing, to show that high intellectual culture is not incompatible with the performance of homely household duties, and that the moral success of which I spoke just now need not be injured, any more than it is in Germany, by intellectual success likewise. I trust that these words may reassure those parents, if any such there be here, who may fear that these lectures will withdraw women from their existing sphere of interest and activity. That they should entertain such a fear is not surprising, after the extravagant opinions and schemes which have been lately broached in various quarters.

The programme to these lectures expressly disclaims any such intentions; and I, as a husband and a father, expressly disclaim any such intention likewise.

"To fit women for the more enlightened performance of their special duties;" to help them towards
learning how to do better what we doubt not they are
already doing well; is, I honestly believe, the only
object of the promoters of this scheme.

Let us see now how some of these special duties can
be better performed by help of a little enlightenment
as to the laws which regulate them.

Now, no man will deny—certainly no man who is
past forty-five, and whose digestion is beginning to
quail before the lumps of beef and mutton which are
the boast of a British kitchen, and to prefer, with Justice Shallow, and, I presume, Sir John Falstaff also,
"any pretty little tiny kickshaws"—no man, I say,
who has reached that age, but will feel it a practical
comfort to him to know that the young ladies of his
family are at all events good cooks; and understand, as
the French do, thrift in the matter of food.

Neither will any parent who wishes, naturally enough,
that his daughters should cost him as little as possible;
and wishes, naturally enough also, that they should be
as well dressed as possible, deny that it would be a
good thing for them to be practical milliners and
mantua-makers; and, by making their own clothes
gracefully and well, exercise thrift in clothing.

But, beside this thrift in clothing, I am not alone,
I believe, in wishing for some thrift in the energy

which produces it. Labour misapplied, you will agree,
is labour wasted; and as dress, I presume, is intended
to adorn the person of the wearer, the making a dress
which only disfigures her may be considered as a
plain case of waste. It would be impertinent in me
to go into any details : but it is impossible to walk
about the streets now without passing young people
who must be under a deep delusion as to the success
of their own toilette. Instead of graceful and noble
simplicity of form, instead of combinations of colour
at once rich and delicate, because in accordance with
the chromatic laws of nature, one meets with phenomena more and more painful to the eye, and startling
to common sense, till one would be hardly more
astonished, and certainly hardly more shocked, if
in a year or two one should pass some one going
about like a Chinese lady, with pinched feet, or
like a savage of the Amazons, with a wooden bung
through her lower lip. It is easy to complain of these
monstrosities : but impossible to cure them, it seems
to me, without an education of the taste, an education
in those laws of nature which produce beauty in form
and beauty in colour. For that the cause of these
failures lies in want of education is patent. They are
most common in—I had almost said they are confined
to—those classes of well-to-do persons who are the
least educated; who have no standard of taste of their

K

own; and who do not acquire any from cultivated friends and relations: who, in consequence, dress themselves blindly according to what they conceive to be the Paris fashions, conveyed at third-hand through an equally uneducated dressmaker; in innocent ignorance of the fact—for fact I believe it to be—that Paris fashions are invented now not in the least for the sake of beauty, but for the sake of producing, through variety, increased expenditure, and thereby increased employment; according to the strange system which now prevails in France of compelling, if not prosperity, at least the signs of it; and like schoolboys before a holiday, nailing up the head of the weather glass to insure fine weather.

Let British ladies educate themselves in those laws of beauty which are as eternal as any other of nature's laws; which may be seen fulfilled, as Mr. Ruskin tells us, so eloquently in every flower and every leaf, in every sweeping down and rippling wave: and they will be able to invent graceful and economical dresses for themselves, without importing tawdry and expensive ugliness from France.

Let me now go a step further, and ask you to consider this.—There are in England now a vast number, and an increasing number, of young women who, from various circumstances which we all know, must in after life be either the mistresses of their own fortunes, or the earners of their own bread. And, to do that wisely and well, they must be more or less women of business; and to be women of business, they must know something of the meaning of the words capital, profit, price, value, labour, wages, and of the relation between those two last. In a word, they must know a little political economy. Nay, I sometimes think that the mistress of every household might find, not only thrift of money, but thrift of brain; freedom from mistakes, anxieties, worries of many kinds, all of which eat out the health as well as the heart, by a little sound knowledge of the principles of political economy.

When we consider that every mistress of a household is continually buying, if not selling; that she is continually hiring and employing labour in the form of servants; and very often, into the bargain, keeping her husband's accounts: I cannot but think that her hard-worked brain might be clearer, and her hard-tried desire to do her duty by every subject in her little kingdom, might be more easily satisfied, had she read something of what Mr. John Stuart Mill has written, especially on the duties of employer and employed. A capitalist, a commercialist, an employer of labour, and an accountant—every mistress of a household is all these, whether she likes it or not; and it would be surely well for her, in so very complicated a state of society as this, not to trust merely to that mother-wit, that intuitive sagacity and innate power of ruling her fellow-creatures, which carries women so nobly through their work in simpler and less civilised societies.

And here I stop to answer those who may say—as I have heard it said—That a woman's intellect is not fit for business ; that when a woman takes to business, she is apt to do it ill, and unpleasantly likewise : to be more suspicious, more irritable, more grasping, more unreasonble, than regular men of business would be : that— as I have heard it put—"a woman does not fight fair." The answer is simple. That a woman's intellect is eminently fitted for business is proved by the enormous amount of business she gets through without any special training for it: but those faults in a woman of which some men complain are simply the results of her not having had a special training. She does not know the laws of business. She does not know the rules of the game she is playing; and therefore she is playing it in the dark, in fear and suspicion, apt to judge of questions on personal grounds, often offending those with whom she has to do, and oftener still making herself miserable over matters of law or of business, on which a little sound knowledge would set her head and her heart at rest.

When I have seen widows, having the care of children, of a great household, of a great estate, of a great business, struggling heroically, and yet often mistakenly;

blamed severely for selfishness and ambition, while they were really sacrificing themselves with the divine instinct of a mother for their children's interest: I have stood by with mingled admiration and pity, and said to myself—"How nobly she is doing the work without teaching! How much more nobly would she have done it had she been taught! She is now doing the work at the most enormous waste of energy and of virtue: had she had knowledge, thrift would have followed it; she would have done more work with far less trouble. She will probably kill herself if she goes on: sound knowledge would have saved her health, saved her heart, saved her friends, and helped the very loved ones for whom she labours, not always with success."

A little political economy, therefore, will at least do no harm to a woman; especially if she have to take care of herself in after life; neither, I think, will she be much harmed by some sound knowledge of another subject, which I see promised in these lectures,—"Natural philosophy, in its various branches, such as the chemistry of common life, light, heat, electricity, &c., &c."

A little knowledge of the laws of light, for instance, would teach many women that by shutting themselves up day after day, week after week, in darkened rooms, they are as certainly committing a waste of health, destroying their vital energy, and diseasing their brains, as if they were taking so much poison the whole time.

A little knowledge of the laws of heat would teach women not to clothe themselves and their children after foolish and insufficient fashions, which in this climate sow the seeds of a dozen different diseases, and have to be atoned for by perpetual anxieties, and by perpetual doctors' bills; and as for a little knowledge of the laws of electricity, one thrift I am sure it would produce—thrift to us men, of having to answer continual inquiries as to what the weather is going to be, when a slight knowledge of the barometer, or of the form of the clouds and the direction of the wind, would enable many a lady to judge for herself, and not, after inquiry on inquiry, disregard all warnings, go out on the first appearance of a strip of blue sky, and come home wet through, with what she calls "only a chill," but which really means a nail driven into her coffin— a probable shortening, though it may be a very small one, of her mortal life; because the food of the next twenty-four hours, which should have gone to keep the vital heat at its normal standard, will have to be wasted in raising it up to that standard, from which it has fallen by a chill.

Ladies; these are subjects on which I must beg to speak a little more at length, premising them by one statement, which may seem jest, but is solemn earnest —that, if the medical men of this or any other city were what the world now calls "alive to their own

interests "—that is, to the mere making of money;
instead of being, what medical men are, the most generous, disinterested, and high-minded class in these
realms, then they would oppose by all means in their
power the delivery of lectures on natural philosophy
to women. For if women act upon what they learn in
those lectures—and having women's hearts, they will
act upon it—there ought to follow a decrease of sickness and an increase of health, especially among
children; a thrift of life, and a thrift of expense
besides, which would very seriously affect the income
of medical men.

For let me ask you, ladies, with all courtesy, but with
all earnestness—Are you aware of certain facts, of
which every one of those excellent medical men is too
well aware? Are you aware that more human beings
are killed in England every year by unnecessary and
preventable diseases than were killed at Waterloo or at
Sadowa? Are you aware that the great majority of
those victims are children? Are you aware that the
diseases which carry them off are for the most part
such as ought to be specially under the control of the
women who love them, pet them, educate them, and
would in many cases, if need be, lay down their lives
for them? Are you aware, again, of the vast amount
of disease which, so both wise mothers and wise doctors
assure me, is engendered in the sleeping-room from

simple ignorance of the laws of ventilation, and in the
school-room likewise, from simple ignorance of the
laws of physiology? from an ignorance of which I
shall mention no other case here save one—that too
often from ignorance of signs of approaching disease, a
child is punished for what is called idleness, listless-
ness, wilfulness, sulkiness; and punished, too, in the
unwisest way—by an increase of tasks and confinement
to the house, thus overtasking still more a brain already
overtasked, and depressing still more, by robbing it of
oxygen and of exercise, a system already depressed?
Are you aware, I ask again, of all this? I speak earnestly upon this point, because I speak with experience.
As a single instance: a medical man, a friend of mine,
passing by his own school-room, heard one of his own
little girls screaming and crying, and went in. The
governess, an excellent woman, but wholly ignorant of
the laws of physiology, complained that the child had
of late become obstinate and would not learn; and that
therefore she must punish her by keeping her indoors
over the unlearnt lessons. The father, who knew that
the child was usually a very good one, looked at her
carefully for a little while; sent her out of the school-
room; and then said, "That child must not open a book
for a month." "If I had not acted so," he said to me,
"I should have had that child dead of brain disease
within the year."

Now, in the face of such facts as these, is it too much to ask of mothers, sisters, aunts, nurses, governesses—all who may be occupied in the care of children, especially of girls—that they should study thrift of human health and human life, by studying somewhat the laws of life and health? There are books—I may say a whole literature of books—written by scientific doctors on these matters, which are in my mind far more important to the schoolroom than half the trashy accomplishments, so-called, which are expected to be known by governesses. But are they bought? Are they even to be bought, from most country booksellers? Ah, for a little knowledge of the laws to the neglect of which is owing so much fearful disease, which, if it does not produce immediate death, too often leaves the constitution impaired for years to come. Ah the waste of health and strength in the young; the waste, too, of anxiety and misery in those who love and tend them. How much of it might be saved by a little rational education in those laws of nature which are the will of God about the welfare of our bodies, and which, therefore, we are as much bound to know and to obey, as we are bound to know and obey the spiritual laws whereon depends the welfare of our souls.

Pardon me, ladies, if I have given a moment's pain to any one here: but I appeal to every medical man in the room whether I have not spoken the truth; and having such an opportunity as this, I felt that I must speak for the sake of children, and of women likewise, or else for ever hereafter hold my peace.

Let me pass on from this painful subject—for painful it has been to me for many years—to a question of intellectual thrift—by which I mean just now thrift of words; thrift of truth; restraint of the tongue; accuracy and modesty in statement.

Mothers complain to me that girls are apt to be—not intentionally untruthful—but exaggerative, prejudiced, incorrect, in repeating a conversation or describing an event; and that from this fault arise, as is to be expected, misunderstandings, quarrels, rumours, slanders, scandals, and what not.

Now, for this waste of words there is but one cure: and if I be told that it is a natural fault of women; that they cannot take the calm judicial view of matters which men boast, and often boast most wrongly, that they can take; that under the influence of hope, fear, delicate antipathy, honest moral indignation, they will let their eyes and ears be governed by their feelings; and see and hear only what they wish to see and hear: I answer, that it is not for me as a man to start such a theory; but that if it be true, it is an additional argument for some education which will correct this supposed natural defect. And I say deliberately that there is but one sort of education which will correct it; one which will teach young women to observe facts accurately, judge them calmly, and describe them carefully, without adding or distorting: and that is, some training in natural science.

I beg you not to be startled: but if you are, then test the truth of my theory by playing to-night at the game called "Russian Scandal;" in which a story, repeated in secret by one player to the other, comes out at the end of the game, owing to the inaccurate and—forgive me if I say it—uneducated brains through which it has passed, utterly unlike its original; not only ludicrously maimed and distorted, but often with the most fantastic additions of events, details, names, dates, places, which each player will aver that he received from the player before him. I am afraid that too much of the average gossip of every city, town, and village is little more than a game of "Russian Scandal;" with this difference, that while one is but a game, the other is but too mischievous earnest.

But now, if among your party there shall be an average lawyer, medical man, or man of science, you will find that he, and perhaps he alone, will be able to retail accurately the story which has been told him. And why? Simply because his mind has been trained to deal with facts; to ascertain exactly what he does see or hear, and to imprint its leading features strongly and clearly on his memory.

Now, you certainly cannot make young ladies barristers or attorneys; nor employ their brains in getting up cases, civil or criminal; and as for chemistry, they and their parents may have a reasonable antipathy to smells, blackened fingers, and occasional explosions and poisonings. But you may make them something of botanists, zoologists, geologists.

I could say much on this point: allow me at least to say this: I verily believe that any young lady who would employ some of her leisure time in collecting wild flowers, carefully examining them, verifying them, and arranging them; or who would in her summer trip to the sea-coast do the same by the common objects of the shore, instead of wasting her holiday, as one sees hundreds doing, in lounging on benches on the esplanade, reading worthless novels, and criticizing dresses —that such a young lady, I say, would not only open her own mind to a world of wonder, beauty, and wisdom, which, if it did not make her a more reverent and pious soul, she cannot be the woman which I take for granted she is; but would save herself from the habit— I had almost said the necessity—of gossip; because she would have things to think of and not merely persons; facts instead of fancies; while she would acquire something of accuracy, of patience, of methodical observation and judgment, which would stand her in good stead in the events of daily life, and increase her power of bridling her tongue and her imagination. "God is in heaven, and thou upon earth; therefore let thy words be few;" is the lesson which those are learning all day long who study the works of God with reverent accuracy, lest by misrepresenting them they should be tempted to say that God has done that which He has not; and in that wholesome discipline I long that women as well as men should share.

And now I come to a thrift of the highest kind, as contrasted with a waste the most deplorable and ruinous of all; thrift of those faculties which connect us with the unseen and spiritual world; with humanity, with Christ, with God; thrift of the immortal spirit. I am not going now to give you a sermon on duty. You hear such, I doubt not, in church every Sunday, far better than I can preach to you. I am going to speak rather of thrift of the heart, thrift of the emotions. How they are wasted in these days in reading what are called sensation novels, all know but too well; how British literature—all that the best hearts and intellects among our forefathers have bequeathed to us—is neglected for light fiction, the reading of which is, as a lady well said, "the worst form of intemperance—dram-drinking and opium-eating, intellectual and moral."

I know that the young will delight—they have delighted in all ages, and will to the end of time—in fictions which deal with that "oldest tale which is for ever new." Novels will be read: but that is all the more reason why women should be trained, by the perusal of a higher, broader, deeper literature, to distinguish the good novel from the bad, the moral from the immoral, the noble from the base, the true work of art from the sham which hides its shallowness and vulgarity under a tangled plot and melodramatic situations. She should learn—and that she can only learn by cultivation—to discern with joy, and drink in with reverence, the good, the beautiful, and the true; and to turn with the fine scorn of a pure and strong womanhood from the bad, the ugly, and the false.

And if any parent should be inclined to reply—"Why lay so much stress upon educating a girl in British literature? Is it not far more important to make our daughters read religious books? I answer—Of course it is. I take for granted that that is done in a Christian land. But I beg you to recollect that there are books and books; and that in these days of a free press it is impossible, in the long run, to prevent girls reading books of very different shades of opinion, and very different religious worth. It may be, therefore, of the very highest importance to a girl to have her intellect, her taste, her emotions, her moral sense, in a word, her whole womanhood, so cultivated and regulated that she shall herself be able to discern the true from the false, the orthodox from the unorthodox, the truly devout from the merely sentimental, the Gospel from its counterfeits.

I should have thought that there never had been in Britain, since the Reformation, a crisis at which young Englishwomen required more careful cultivation on these matters; if at least they are to be saved from making themselves and their families miserable; and from ending—as I have known too many end—with broken hearts, broken brains, broken health, and an early grave.

Take warning by what you see abroad. In every country where the women are uneducated, unoccupied; where their only literature is French novels or translations of them—in every one of those countries the women, even to the highest, are the slaves of superstition, and the puppets of priests. In proportion as, in certain other countries—notably, I will say, in Scotland—the women are highly educated, family life and family secrets are sacred, and the woman owns allegiance and devotion to no confessor or director, but to her own husband or to her own family.

I say plainly, that if any parents wish their daughters to succumb at last to some quackery or superstition, whether calling itself scientific, or calling itself religious—and there are too many of both just now—they cannot more certainly effect their purpose than by allowing her to grow up ignorant, frivolous, luxurious, vain; with her emotions excited, but not satisfied, by the reading of foolish and even immoral novels.

In such a case the more delicate and graceful the organization, the more noble and earnest the nature, which has been neglected, the more certain it is—I know too well what I am saying—to go astray.

The time of depression, disappointment, vacuity, all but despair, must come. The immortal spirit, finding no healthy satisfaction for its highest aspirations, is but too likely to betake itself to an unhealthy and exciting superstition. Ashamed of its own long self-indulgence, it is but too likely to flee from itself into a morbid asceticism. Not having been taught its God-given and natural duties in the world, it is but too likely to betake itself, from the mere craving for action, to self-invented and unnatural duties out of the world. Ignorant of true science, yet craving to understand the wonders of nature and of spirit, it is but too likely to betake itself to non-science—nonsense as it is usually called—whether of spirit-rapping and mesmerism, or of miraculous relics and winking pictures. Longing for guidance and teaching, and never having been taught to guide and teach itself, it is but too likely to deliver itself up in self-despair to the guidance and teaching of those who, whether they be quacks or fanatics, look on uneducated women as their natural prey.

You will see, I am sure, from what I have said, that

it is not my wish that you should become mere learned women; mere female pedants, as useless and unpleasing as male pedants are wont to be. The education which I set before you is not to be got by mere hearing lectures or reading books: for it is an education of your whole character; a self-education; which really means a committing of yourself to God, that He may educate you. Hearing lectures is good, for it will teach you how much there is to be known, and how little you know. Reading books is good, for it will give you habits of regular and diligent study. And therefore I urge on you strongly private study, especially in case a library should be formed here of books on those most practical subjects of which I have been speaking. But, after all, both lectures and books are good, mainly in as far as they furnish matter for reflection: while the desire to reflect and the ability to reflect must come, as I believe, from above. The honest craving after light and power, after knowledge, wisdom, active usefulness, must come—and may it come to you—by the inspiration of the Spirit of God.

One word more, and I have done. Let me ask women to educate themselves, not for their own sakes merely, but for the sake of others. For, whether they will or not, they must educate others. I do not speak merely of those who may be engaged in the work of direct teaching; that they ought to be well taught them-

L

selves, who can doubt? I speak of those—and in so doing I speak of every woman, young and old—who exercises as wife, as mother, as aunt, as sister, or as friend, an influence, indirect it may be, and unconscious, but still potent and practical, on the minds and characters of those about them, especially of men. How potent and practical that influence is, those know best who know most of the world and most of human nature. There are those who consider—and I agree with them—that the education of boys under the age of twelve years ought to be entrusted as much as possible to women. Let me ask—of what period of youth and of manhood does not the same hold true? I pity the ignorance and conceit of the man who fancies that he has nothing left to learn from cultivated women. I should have thought that the very mission of woman was to be, in the highest sense, the educator of man from infancy to old age; that that was the work towards which all the God-given capacities of women pointed; for which they were to be educated to the highest pitch. I should have thought that it was the glory of woman that she was sent into the world to live for others, rather than for herself; and therefore I should say—Let her smallest rights be respected, her smallest wrongs redressed: but let her never be persuaded to forget that she is sent into the world to teach man—what, I believe, she has been teaching him all along, even in the savage state—namely, that there is something more necessary than the claiming of rights, and that is, the performing of duties; to teach him specially, in these so-called intellectual days, that there is something more than intellect, and that is—purity and virtue. Let her never be persuaded to forget that her calling is not the lower and more earthly one of self-assertion, but the higher and the diviner calling of self-sacrifice; and let her never desert that higher life, which lives in others and for others, like her Redeemer and her Lord.

And if any should answer that this doctrine would keep· woman a dependant and a slave, I rejoin—Not so: it would keep her what she should be—the mistress of all around her, because mistress of herself. And more, I should express a fear that those who made that answer had not yet seen into the mystery of true greatness and true strength; that they did not yet understand the true magnanimity, the true royalty of that spirit, by which the Son of man came not to be ministered unto, but to minister, and to give His life a ransom for many.

Surely that is woman's calling—to teach man: and to teach him what? To teach him, after all, that his calling is the same as hers, if he will but see the things which belong to his peace. To temper his fiercer, coarser, more self-assertive nature, by the contact of

her gentleness, purity, self-sacrifice. To make him see
that not by blare of trumpets, not by noise, wrath,
greed, ambition, intrigue, puffery, is good and lasting
work to be done on earth: but by wise self-distrust,
by silent labour, by lofty self-control, by that charity
which hopeth all things, believeth all things, endureth
all things; by such an example, in short, as women
now in tens of thousands set to those around them;
such as they will show more and more, the more their
whole womanhood is educated to employ its powers
without waste and without haste in harmonious unity.
Let the woman begin in girlhood, if such be her happy
lot—to quote the words of a great poet, a great philosopher, and a great Churchman, William Wordsworth—
let her begin, I say—

> " With all things round about her drawn
> From May-time and the cheerful dawn ;
> A dancing shape, an image gay,
> To haunt, to startle, and waylay."

Let her develop onwards—

> " A spirit, yet a woman too,
> With household motions light and free,
> And steps of virgin liberty.
> A countenance in which shall meet
> Sweet records, promises as sweet ;
> A creature not too bright and good
> For human nature's daily food ;
> For transient sorrows, simple wiles,
> Praise, blame, love, kisses, tears, and smiles.

But let her highest and her final development be that

which not nature, but self-education alone can bring—
that which makes her once and for ever—

> " A being breathing thoughtful breath ;
> A traveller betwixt life and death.
> With reason firm, with temperate will,
> Endurance, foresight, strength and skill.
> A perfect woman, nobly planned,
> To warn, to comfort and command.
> And yet a spirit still and bright
> With something of an angel light."

THE STUDY OF NATURAL HISTORY.

A LECTURE DELIVERED TO THE OFFICERS OF THE ROYAL
ARTILLERY, WOOLWICH.

GENTLEMEN :—When I accepted the honour of lecturing
here, I took for granted that so select an audience
would expect from me not mere amusement, but somewhat of instruction ; or, if that be too ambitious a word
for me to use, at least some fresh hint—if I were able
to give one—as to how they should fulfil the ideal of
military men in such an age as this.

To touch on military matters, even had I been con-
versant with them, seemed to me an impertinence. I
am bound to take for granted that every man knows
his own business best ; and I incline more and more to
the opinion that military men should be left to work
out the problems of their art for themselves, without
the advice or criticism of civilians. But I hold—and I
am sure that you will agree with me—that if the soldier
is to be thus trusted by the nation, and left to himself
to do his own work his own way, he must be educated

in all practical matters as highly as the average of educated civilians. He must know all that they know, and his own art besides. Just as a clergyman, being a man plus a priest, is bound to be a man, and a good man, over and above his priesthood, so is the soldier bound to be a civilian, and a highly-educated civilian, plus his soldierly qualities and acquirements.

It seemed to me, therefore, that I might, without impertinence, ask you to consider a branch of knowledge which is becoming yearly more and more important in the eyes of well-educated civilians; of which, therefore, the soldier ought at least to know something, in order to put him on a par with the general intelligence of the nation. I do not say that he is to devote much time to it, or to follow it up into specialities: but that he ought to be well grounded in its principles and methods; that he ought to be aware of its importance and its usefulness; that so, if he comes into contact—as he will more and more—with scientific men, he may understand them, respect them, befriend them, and be befriended by them in turn; and how desirable this last result is, I shall tell you hereafter.

There are those, I doubt not, among my audience who do not need the advice which I shall presume to give to-night; who belong to that fast increasing class among officers of whom I have often said—and I have found scientific men cordially agree with me—that they are the most modest and the most teachable of men. But even in their case there can be no harm in going over deliberately a question of such importance; in putting it, as it were, into shape; and insisting on arguments which may perhaps not have occurred to some of them.

Let me, in the first place, reassure those—if any such there be—who may suppose, from the title of my lecture, that I am only going to recommend them to collect weeds and butterflies, "rats and mice, and such small deer." Far from it. The honourable title of Natural History has, and unwisely, been restricted too much of late years to the mere study of plants and animals. I desire to restore the words to their original and proper meaning—the History of Nature; that is, of all that is born, and grows in time; in short, of all natural objects.

If any one shall say—By that definition you make not only geology and chemistry branches of natural history, but meteorology and astronomy likewise—I cannot deny it. They deal, each of them, with realms of Nature. Geology is, literally, the natural history of soils and lands; chemistry the natural history of compounds, organic and inorganic; meteorology the natural history of climates; astronomy the natural history of planetary and solar bodies. And more, you cannot

now study deeply any branch of what is popularly
called Natural History—that is, plants and animals—
without finding it necessary to learn something, and
more and more as you go deeper, of those very sciences.
As the marvellous interdependence of all natural objects
and forces unfolds itself more and more, so the once
separate sciences, which treated of different classes of
natural objects, are forced to interpenetrate, as it were ;
and to supplement themselves by knowledge borrowed
from each other. Thus—to give a single instance—no
man can now be a first-rate botanist unless he be also
no mean meteorologist, no mean geologist, and—as Mr.
Darwin has shown in his extraordinary discoveries
about the fertilisation of plants by insects—no mean
entomologist likewise.

It is difficult, therefore, and indeed somewhat unwise
and unfair, to put any limit to the term Natural History, save that it shall deal only with nature and with
matter ; and shall not pretend—as some would have it
to do just now—to go out of its own sphere to meddle
with moral and spiritual matters. But, for practical
purposes, we may define the natural history of any
given spot as the history of the causes which have
made it what it is, and filled it with the natural objects
which it holds. And if any one would know how to
study the natural history of a place, and how to write
it, let him read—and if he has read its delightful pages

in youth, read once again—that hitherto unrivalled little
monograph, White's 'Natural History of Selborne;' and
let him then try, by the light of improved science, to
do for any district where he may be stationed, what
White did for Selborne nearly one hundred years ago.
Let him study its plants, its animals, its soils and
rocks; and last, but not least, its scenery, as the total
outcome of what the soils, and plants, and animals
have made it. I say, have made it. How far the
nature of the soils and the rocks will affect the scenery
of a district may be well learnt from a very clever
and interesting little book of Professor Geikie's, on
'The Scenery of Scotland as affected by its Geological
Structure.' How far the plants, and trees affect not
merely the general beauty, the richness or barrenness
of a country, but also its very shape; the rate at which
the hills are destroyed and washed into the lowland;
the rate at which the seaboard is being removed by the
action of waves—all these are branches of study which
is becoming more and more important.

And even in the study of animals and their effects on
the vegetation, questions of really deep interest will
arise. You will find that certain plants and trees
cannot thrive in a district, while others can, because
the former are browsed down by cattle, or their seeds
eaten by birds, and the latter are not; that certain
seeds are carried in the coats of animals, or wafted

abroad by winds—others are not; certain trees destroyed wholesale by insects, while others are not;
that in a hundred ways the animal and vegetable life
of a district act and react upon each other, and that
the climate, the average temperature, the maximum
and minimum temperatures, the rainfall, act on them,
and in the case of the vegetation, are reacted on again
by them. The diminution of rainfall by the destruction
of forests, its increase by replanting them, and the
effect of both on the healthiness or unhealthiness of a
place—as in the case of the Mauritius, where a once
healthy island has become pestilential, seemingly from
the clearing away of the vegetation on the banks of
streams—all this, though to study it deeply requires a
fair knowledge of meteorology, and even of a science or
two more, is surely well worth the attention of any
educated man who is put in charge of the health and
lives of human beings.

You will surely agree with me that the habit of
mind required for such a study as this, is the very
same as is required for successful military study. In
fact, I should say that the same intellect which would
develop into a great military man, would develop also
into a great naturalist. I say, intellect. The military
man would require—what the naturalist would not—
over and above his intellect, a special force of will, in
order to translate his theories into fact, and make his

campaigns in the field and not merely on paper. But I am speaking only of the habit of mind required for study; of that inductive habit of mind which works, steadily and by rule, from the known to the unknown : that habit of mind of which it has been said :—" The habit of seeing; the habit of knowing what we see; the habit of discerning differences and likenesses; the habit of classifying accordingly; the habit of searching for hypotheses which shall connect and explain those classified facts; the habit of verifying these hypotheses by applying them to fresh facts; the habit of throwing them away bravely if they will not fit; the habit of general patience, diligence, accuracy, reverence for facts for their own sake, and love of truth for its own sake; in one word, the habit of reverent and implicit obedience to the laws of Nature, whatever they may be —these are not merely intellectual, but also moral habits, which will stand men in practical good stead in every affair of life, and in every question, even the most awful, which may come before them as rational and social beings." And specially valuable are they, surely, to the military man, the very essence of whose study, to be successful, lies first in continuous and accurate observation, and then in calm and judicious arrangement.

Therefore it is that I hold, and hold strongly, that the study of physical science, far from interfering with an officer's studies, much less unfitting for them, must assist him in them, by keeping his mind always in the very attitude and the very temper which they require.

If any smile at this theory of mine, let them recollect one curious fact: that perhaps the greatest captain of the old world was trained by perhaps the greatest philosopher of the old world—the father of Natural History; that Aristotle was the tutor of Alexander of Macedon. I do not fancy, of course, that Aristotle taught Alexander any Natural History. But this we know, that he taught him to use those very faculties by which Aristotle became a natural historian, and many things beside; that he called out in his pupil somewhat of his own extraordinary powers of observation, extraordinary powers of arrangement. He helped to make him a great general: but he helped to make him more—a great politician, coloniser, discoverer. He instilled into him such a sense of the importance of Natural History, that Alexander helped him nobly in his researches; and, if Athenæus is to be believed, gave him 800 talents towards perfecting his history of animals. Surely it is not too much to say that this close friendship between the natural philosopher and the soldier has changed the whole course of civilisation to this very day. Do not consider me Utopian when I tell you, that I should like to see the study of physical science an integral part of the curriculum of every military school. I would train the mind of the lad who was to become hereafter an officer in the army—and in the navy likewise—by accustoming him to careful observation of, and sound thought about, the face of nature; of the commonest objects under his feet, just as much as of the stars above his head; provided always that he learnt, not at second-hand from books, but where alone he can really learn either war or nature—in the field; by actual observation, actual experiment. A laboratory for chemical experiment is a good thing, it is true, as far as it goes; but I should prefer to the laboratory a naturalists' field club, such as are prospering now at several of the best public schools, certain that the boys would get more of sound inductive habits of mind, as well as more health, manliness, and cheerfulness, amid scenes to remember which will be a joy for ever, than they ever can by bending over retorts and crucibles, amid smells even to remember which is a pain for ever.

But I would, whether a field club existed or not, require of every young man entering the army or navy —indeed of every young man entering any liberal profession whatsoever—a fair knowledge, such as would enable him to pass an examination, in what the Germans call *Erd-kunde*—earth-lore—in that knowledge of the face of the earth and of its products, for which we English have as yet cared so little that we

have actually no English name for it, save the clumsy
and questionable one of physical geography; and, I
am sorry to say, hardly any readable school books
about it, save Keith Johnston's 'Physical Atlas'—an
acquaintance with which last I should certainly require
of young men.

It does seem most strange—or rather will seem most
strange 100 years hence—that we, the nation of
colonists, the nation of sailors, the nation of foreign
commerce, the nation of foreign military stations, the
nation of travellers for travelling's sake, the nation of
which one man here and another there—as Schleiden
sets forth in his book, 'The Plant,' in a charming
ideal conversation at the Travellers' Club—has seen
and enjoyed more of the wonders and beauties of this
planet than the men of any nation, not even excepting
the Germans—that this nation, I say, should as yet
have done nothing, or all but nothing, to teach in her
schools a knowledge of that planet, of which she needs
to know more, and can if she will know more, than any
other nation upon it.

As for the practical utility of such studies to a soldier,
I only need, I trust, to hint at it to such an assembly
as this. All must see of what advantage a rough knowledge of the botany of a district would be to an officer
leading an exploring party, or engaged in bush warfare.
To know what plants are poisonous; what plants, too,

are eatable—and many more are eatable than is usually
supposed; what plants yield oleaginous substances,
whether for food or for other uses; what plants yield
vegetable acids, as preventives of scurvy; what timbers
are available for each of many different purposes; what
will resist wet, salt-water, and the attacks of insects;
what, again, can be used, at a pinch, for medicine or for
styptics—and be sure, as a wise West Indian doctor
once said to me, that there is more good medicine wild
in the bush than there is in all the druggists' shops—
surely all this is a knowledge not beneath the notice
of any enterprising officer, above all of an officer of
engineers. I only ask any one who thinks that I may
be in the right, to glance through the lists of useful
vegetable products given in Lindley's ' Vegetable Kingdom '—a miracle of learning—and see the vast field
open still to a thoughtful and observant man, even
while on service; and not to forget that such knowledge, if he should hereafter leave the service and settle,
as many do, in a distant land, may be a solid help to
his future prosperity. So strongly do I feel on this
matter, that I should like to see some knowledge at
least of Dr. Oliver's excellent little ' First Book of
Indian Botany' required of all officers going to our
Indian Empire: but as that will not be, at least for
many a year to come, I recommend any gentlemen
going to India to get that book, and wile away the

hours of the outward voyage by acquiring knowledge which will be a continual source of interest, and it may be now and then of profit, to them during their stay abroad.

And for geology, again. As I do not expect you all, or perhaps any of you, to become such botanists as General Monro, whose recent 'Monograph of the Bamboos' is an honour to British botanists, and a proof of the scientific power which is to be found here and there among British officers: so I do not expect you to become such geologists as Sir Roderick Murchison, or even to add such a grand chapter to the history of extinct animals as Major Cautley did by his discoveries in the Sewalik Hills. Nevertheless, you can learn— and I should earnestly advise you to learn—geology and mineralogy enough to be of great use to you in your profession, and of use, too, should you relinquish your profession hereafter. It must be profitable for any man, and specially for you, to know how and where to find good limestone, building stone, road metal; it must be good to be able to distinguish ores and mineral products; it must be good to know—as a geologist will usually know, even in a country which he sees for the first time—where water is likely to be found, and at what probable depth; it must be good to know whether the water is fit for drinking or not, whether it is unwholesome or merely muddy; it must be good to

M

know what spots are likely to be healthy, and what
unhealthy, for encamping.   The two last questions
depend, doubtless, on meteorological as well as geological accidents : but the answers to them will be most
surely found out by the scientific man, because the facts
connected with them are, like all other facts, determined
by natural laws.   After what one has heard, in past
years, of barracks built in spots plainly pestilential;
of soldiers encamped in ruined cities, reeking with the
dirt and poison of centuries ; of—but it is not my
place to find fault; all I will say is, that the wise and
humane officer, when once his eyes are opened to the
practical value of physical science, will surely try to
acquaint himself somewhat with those laws of drainage
and of climate, geological, meteorological, chemical,
which influence, often with terrible suddenness and
fury, the health of whole armies.   He will not find it
beyond his province to ascertain the amount and period
of rainfalls, the maxima of heat and of cold which his
troops may have to endure, and many another point
on which their health and efficiency—nay, their very
life may depend, but which are now too exclusively
delegated to the doctor, to whose province they do not
really belong.   For cure, I take the liberty of believing,
is the duty of the medical officer; prevention, that of
the military.

Thus much I can say just now—and there is much more

to be said—on the practical uses of the study of Natural
History. But let me remind you, on the other side, if
Natural History will help you, you in return can help
her; and would, I doubt not, help her, and help
scientific men at home, if once you looked fairly and
steadily at the immense importance of Natural History
—of the knowledge of the "face of the earth." I
believe that all will one day feel, more or less, that to
know the earth *on* which we live, and the laws of it *by*
which we live, is a sacred duty to ourselves, to our
children after us, and to all whom we may have to
command and to influence; aye, and a duty to God
likewise. For is it not a duty of common reverence and
faith towards Him, if He has put us into a beautiful
and wonderful place, and given us faculties by which
we can see, and enjoy, and use that place—is it not a
duty of reverence and faith towards Him to use these
faculties, and to learn the lessons which He has laid open
for us? If you feel that, as I think you all will some
day feel, then you will surely feel likewise that it will
be a good deed—I do not say a necessary duty, but
still a good deed and praiseworthy—to help physical
science forward; and to add your contributions, however
small, to our general knowledge of the earth. And
how much may be done for science by British officers,
especially on foreign stations, I need not point out. I
know that much has been done, chivalrously and well,

by officers; and that men of science owe them, and
give them, hearty thanks for their labours. But I should
like, I confess, to see more done still. I should like to
see every foreign station, what one or two highly-
educated officers might easily make it, an advanced post
of physical science, in regular communication with our
scientific societies at home, sending to them accurate
and methodic details of the natural history of each
district—details $\frac{99}{100}$ths of which might seem worthless
in the eyes of the public, but which would all be
precious in the eyes of scientific men, who know that
no fact is really unimportant; and more, that while
plodding patiently through seemingly unimportant
facts, you may stumble on one of infinite importance,
both scientific and practical. For the student of nature,
gentlemen, if he will be but patient, diligent, methodical, is liable at any moment to the same good fortune
as befel Saul of old, when he went out to seek his father's
asses, and found a kingdom.

There are those, lastly, who have neither time nor
taste for the technicalities, and nice distinctions, of
formal Natural History; who enjoy Nature, but as
artists or as sportsmen, and not as men of science.
Let them follow their bent freely: but let them not
suppose that in following it they can do nothing towards enlarging our knowledge of Nature, especially
when on foreign stations. So far from it, drawings

ought always to be valuable, whether of plants, animals, or scenery, provided only they are accurate; and the more spirited and full of genius they are, the more accurate they are certain to be; for Nature being alive, a lifeless copy of her is necessarily an untrue copy. Most thankful to any officer for a mere sight of sketches will be the closet botanist, who, to his own sorrow, knows three-fourths of his plants only from dried specimens; or the closet zoologist, who knows his animals from skins and bones. And if any one answers—But I cannot draw. I rejoin, You can at least photograph. If a young officer, going out to foreign parts, and knowing nothing at all about physical science, did me the honour to ask me what he could do for science, I should tell him—Learn to photograph; take photographs of every strange bit of rock-formation which strikes your fancy, and of every widely extended view which may give a notion of the general lie of the country. Append, if you can, a note or two, saying whether a plain is rich or barren; whether the rock is sandstone, limestone, granitic, metamorphic, or volcanic lava; and if there be more rocks than one, which of them lies on the other; and send them to be exhibited at a meeting of the Geological Society. I doubt not that the learned gentlemen there will find in your photographs a valuable hint or two, for which they will be much obliged. I learnt, for instance, what seemed to me most valuable geological lessons, from mere glances at drawings—I believe from photographs —of the Abyssinian ranges about Magdala.

Or again, let a man, if he knows nothing of botany, not trouble himself with collecting and drying specimens ; let him simply photograph every strange and new tree or plant he sees, to give a general notion of its species, its look ; let him append, where he can, a photograph of its leafage, flower, fruit ; and send them to Dr. Hooker, or any distinguished botanist : and he will find that, though he may know nothing of botany, he will have pretty certainly increased the knowledge of those who do know.

The sportsman, again—I mean the sportsman of that type which seems peculiar to these islands, who loves toil and danger for their own sakes ; he surely is a naturalist, ipso facto, though he knows it not. He has those very habits of keen observation on which all sound knowledge of nature is based ; and he, if he will —as he may do without interfering with his sport— can study the habits of the animals among whom he spends wholesome and exciting days. You have only to look over such good old books as Williams's 'Wild Sports of the East,' Campbell's 'Old Forest Ranger,' Lloyd's 'Scandinavian Adventures,' and last, but not least, Waterton's 'Wanderings,' to see what valuable additions to true zoology—the knowledge of live creatures, not merely dead ones—British sportsmen have made, and still can make. And as for the employment of time, which often hangs so heavily on a soldier's hands, really I am ready to say, if you are neither men of science, nor draughtsmen, nor sportsmen, why go and collect beetles. It is not very dignified, I know, nor exciting: but it will be something to do. It cannot harm you, if you take, as beetle-hunters do, an india-rubber sheet to lie on; and it will certainly benefit science. Moreover, there will be a noble humility in the act. You will confess to the public that you consider yourself only fit to catch beetles; by which very confession you will prove yourself fit for much finer things than catching beetles; and meanwhile, as I said before, you will be at least out of harm's way. At a foreign barrack once, the happiest officer I met, because the most regularly employed, was one who spent his time in collecting butterflies. He knew nothing about them scientifically—not even their names. He took them simply for their wonderful beauty and variety; and in the hope, too—in which he was really scientific—that if he carefully kept every form which he saw, his collection might be of use some day to entomologists at home. A most pleasant gentleman he was; and, I doubt not, none the worse soldier for his butterfly catching. Commendable, also, in my eyes, was another officer—whom I have not the pleasure of knowing—who, on a remote foreign station, used wisely to escape from the temptations of the world into an entirely original and most pleasant hermitage. For finding—so the story went—that many of the finest insects kept to the tree-tops, and never came to ground at all, he used to settle himself among the boughs of some tree in the tropic forests, with a long-handled net and plenty of cigars, and pass his hours in that airy flower garden, making dashes every now and then at some splendid monster as it fluttered round his head. His example need not be followed by every one; but it must be allowed that —at least as long as he was in his tree—he was neither dawdling, grumbling, spending money, nor otherwise harming himself, and perhaps his fellow creatures, from sheer want of employment.

One word more, and I have done. If I was allowed to give one special piece of advice to a young officer, whether of the army or navy, I would say—Respect scientific men; associate with them; learn from them; find them to be, as you will usually, the most pleasant and instructive of companions: but always respect them. Allow them chivalrously, you who have an acknowledged rank, their yet unacknowledged rank; and treat them as all the world will treat them, in a higher and truer state of civilisation. They do not yet wear the Queen's uniform; they are not yet accepted servants of the State; as they will be in some more perfectly organised and civilised land : but they are soldiers nevertheless, and good soldiers and chivalrous, fighting their nation's battle, often on even less pay than you, and with still less chance of promotion and of fame, against most real and fatal enemies—against ignorance of the laws of this planet, and all the miseries which that ignorance begets. Honour them for their work; sympathise in it; give them a helping hand in it whenever you have an opportunity—and what opportunities you have, I have been trying to sketch for you to-night; and more, work at it yourselves whenever and wherever you can. Show them that the spirit which animates them—the hatred of ignorance and disorder, and of their bestial consequences—animates you likewise; show them that the habit of mind which they value in themselves—the habit of accurate observation and careful judgment—is your habit likewise; show them that you value science, not merely because it gives better weapons of destruction and of defence, but because it helps you to become clear-headed, large-minded, able to take a just and accurate view of any subject which comes before you, and to cast away every old prejudice and every hasty judgment in the face of truth and of duty : and it will be better for you and for them.

But why? What need for the soldier and the man of science to fraternise just now? This need :—The two

classes which will have an increasing, it may be a pre-
ponderating, influence on the fate of the human race
for some time, will be the pupils of Aristotle and those
of Alexander—the men of science and the soldiers.   In
spite of all appearances, and all declamations to the
contrary, that is my firm conviction.   They, and they
alone, will be left to rule ; because they alone, each in
his own sphere, have learnt to obey.   It is therefore
most needful for the welfare of society that they should
pull with, and not against each other ; that they
should understand each other, respect each other, take
counsel with each other, supplement each other's defects, bring out each other's higher tendencies, coun-
teract each other's lower ones.   The scientific man has
something to learn of you, gentlemen, which I doubt
not that he will learn in good time.   You, again, have—as
I have been hinting to you to-night—something to learn
of him, which you, I doubt not, will learn in good time
likewise.   Repeat, each of you according to his powers,
the old friendship between Aristotle and Alexander ;
and so, from the sympathy and co-operation of you
two, a class of thinkers and actors may yet arise which
can save this nation, and the other civilised nations
of the world, from that of which I had rather not
speak ; and wish that I did not think, too often and too
earnestly.

   I may be a dreamer: and I may consider, in my turn,

as wilder dreamers than myself, certain persons who fancy that their only business in life is to make money, the scientific man's only business is to show them how to make money, and the soldier's only business to guard their money for them. Be that as it may, the finest type of civilised man which we are likely to see for some generations to come, will be produced by a combination of the truly military with the truly scientific man. I say—I may be a dreamer: but you at least, as well as my scientific friends, will bear with me; for my dream is to your honour.

ON BIO-GEOLOGY.

An Address given to the Scientific Society of
Winchester.

———◆———

I AM not sure that the subject of my address is rightly
chosen. I am not sure that I ought not to have post-
poned a question of mere natural history, to speak to
you, as scientific men, on the questions of life and
death, which have been forced upon us by the awful
warning of an illustrious personage's illness; of pre-
ventible disease, its frightful prevalency; of the
200,000 persons who are said to have died of fever
alone since the Prince Consort's death, ten years ago ;
of the remedies ; of drainage; of sewage disinfection and
utilisation ; and of the assistance which you, as a body
of scientific men, can give to any effort towards saving
the lives and health of our fellow-citizens from those
unseen poisons which lurk like wild beasts couched in
the jungle, ready to spring at any moment on the un-
suspecting, the innocent, the helpless. Of all this
I longed to speak: but I thought it best only to hint
at it, and leave the question to your common sense and

your humanity; taking for granted that your minds, like the minds of all right-minded Englishmen, have been of late painfully awakened to its importance. It seemed to me almost an impertinence to say more in a city of whose local circumstances I know little or nothing. As an old sanitary reformer, practical, as well as theoretical, I am but too well aware of the difficulties which beset any complete scheme of drainage, especially in an ancient city like this; where men are paying the penalty of their predecessors' ignorance; and dwelling, whether they choose or not, over fifteen centuries of accumulated dirt.

And, therefore, taking for granted that there is energy and intellect enough in Winchester to conquer these difficulties in due time, I go on to ask you to consider, for a time, a subject which is growing more and more important and interesting, a subject the study of which will do much towards raising the field naturalist from a mere collector of specimens—as he was twenty years ago—to a philosopher elucidating some of the grandest problems. I mean the infant science of Bio-geology—the science which treats of the distribution of plants and animals over the globe, and the causes of that distribution.

I doubt not that there are many here who know far more about the subject than I; who are far better read than I am in the works of Forbes, Darwin, Wallace,

Hooker, Moritz Wagner, and the other illustrious men who have written on it. But I may, perhaps, give a few hints which will be of use to the younger members of this Society, and will point out to them how to get a new relish for the pursuit of field science.

Bio-geology, then, begins with asking every plant or animal you meet, large or small, not merely— What is your name? That is the collector and classifier's duty; and a most necessary duty it is, and one to be performed with the most conscientious patience and accuracy, so that a sound foundation may be built for future speculations. But young naturalists should act not merely as Nature's registrars and census-takers, but as her policemen and gamekeepers; and ask everything they meet—How did you get here? By what road did you come? What was your last place of abode? And now you are here, how do you get your living? Are you and your children thriving, like decent people who can take care of themselves, or growing pauperised and degraded, and dying out? Not that we have a fear of your becoming a dangerous class. Madam Nature allows no dangerous classes, in the modern sense. She has, doubtless for some wise reason, no mercy for the weak. She rewards each organism according to its works; and if anything grows too weak or stupid to take care of itself, she gives it its due deserts by letting it die and disappear. So, you plant or you animal, are you among the strong, the successful, the multiplying, the colonising? Or are you among the weak, the failing, the dwindling, the doomed?

These questions may seem somewhat rude: but you may comfort yourself by the thought that plants and animals, though they deserve all kindness, all admiration, deserve no courtesy—at least in this respect. For they are, one and all, wherever you find them, vagrants and landloupers, intruders and conquerors, who have got where they happen to be simply by the law of the strongest—generally not without a little robbery and murder. They have no right save that of possession; the same by which the puffin turns out the old rabbits, eats the young ones, and then lays her eggs in the rabbit burrow—simply because she can.

Now, you will see at once that such a course of questioning will call out a great many curious and interesting answers, if you can only get the things to tell you their story; as you always may, if you will cross-examine them long enough; and will lead you into many subjects beside mere botany or entomology. So various, indeed, are the subjects which you will thus start, that I can only hint at them now in the most cursory fashion.

At the outset you will soon find yourself involved in chemical and meteorological questions: as, for instance, when you ask—How is it that I find one flora on the

sea-shore, another on the sandstone, another on the
chalk, and another on the peat-making gravelly strata?
The usual answer would be, I presume—if we could
work it out by twenty years' experiment, such as Mr.
Lawes, of Rothampsted, has been making on the growth
of grasses and leguminous plants in different soils and
under different manures—the usual answer, I say, would
be—Because we plants want such and such mineral
constituents in our woody fibre; again, because we
want a certain amount of moisture at a certain period
of the year: or, perhaps, simply because the mechanical
arrangement of the particles of a certain soil happens
to suit the shape of our roots and of their stomata.
Sometimes you will get an answer quickly enough;
sometimes not. If you ask, for instance, *Asplenium
viride* how it contrives to grow plentifully in the
Craven of Yorkshire down to 600 or 800 feet above
the sea, while in Snowdon it dislikes growing lower
than 2000 feet, and is not plentiful even there?—it
will reply—Because in the Craven I can get as much
carbonic acid as I want from the decomposing limestone: while on the Snowdon Silurian I get very little;
and I have to make it up by clinging to the mountain
tops, for the sake of the greater rainfall. But if you
ask *Polypodium calcareum*—How is it you choose only
to grow on limestone, while *Polypodium Dryopteris*, of
which, I suspect, you are only a variety, is ready to

grow anywhere?—*Polypodium calcareum* will refuse, as yet, to answer a word.

Again—I can only give you the merest string of hints—you will find in your questionings that many plants and animals have no reason at all to show why they should be in one place and not in another, save the very sound reason for the latter which was suggested to me once by a great naturalist. I was asking— Why don't I find such and such a species in my parish, while it is plentiful a few miles off in exactly the same soil?—and he answered—For the same reason that you are not in America. Because you have not got there. Which answer threw to me a flood of light on this whole science. Things are often where they are, simply because they happen to have got there, and not elsewhere. But they must have got there by some means: and those means I want young naturalists to discover; at least to guess at.

A species, for instance—and I suspect it is a common case with insects—may abound in a single spot, simply because, long years ago, a single brood of eggs happened to hatch at a time when eggs of other species, who would have competed against them for food, did not hatch; and they may remain confined to that spot, though there is plenty of good food for them outside it, simply because they do not increase fast enough to require to spread out in search of more food. Thus I

N

should explain a case which I heard of lately of *Antho-cera trifolii*, abundant for years in one corner of a certain field, and only there; while there was just as much trefoil all round for its larvæ as there was in the selected spot.   I can, I say, only give hints: but they will suffice, I hope, to show the path of thought into which I want young naturalists to turn their minds.

Or, again, you will have to inquire whether the species has not been prevented from spreading by some natural barrier.   Mr. Wallace, whom you all of course know, has shown in his 'Malay Archipelago' that a strait of deep sea can act as such a barrier between species. Moritz Wagner has shown that, in the case of insects, a moderately broad river may divide two closely allied species of beetles, or a very narrow snow-range two closely allied species of moths.

Again, another cause, and a most common one is: that the plants cannot spread because they find the ground beyond them already occupied by other plants, who will not tolerate a fresh mouth, having only just enough to feed themselves.   Take the case of *Saxifraga hypnoides* and *S. umbrosa*, "London pride."   They are two especially strong species.   They show that, *S. hyp-noides* especially, by their power of sporting, of diverging into varieties; they show it equally by their power of thriving anywhere, if they can only get there.   They will both grow in my sandy garden, under a rainfall of only 23 inches, more luxuriantly than in their native mountains under a rainfall of 50 or 60 inches. Then how is it that *S. hypnoides* cannot get down off the mountains; and that *S. umbrosa*, though in Kerry it has got off the mountains and down to the sea level, exterminating, I suspect, many species in its progress, yet cannot get across county Cork? The only answer is, I believe: that both species are continually trying to go ahead; but that the other plants already in front of them are too strong for them, and massacre their infants as soon as born.

And this brings us to another curious question: the sudden and abundant appearance of plants, like the foxglove and *Epilobium angustifolium*, in spots where they have never been seen before. Are their seeds, as some think, dormant in the ground; or are the seeds which have germinated fresh ones wafted thither by wind or otherwise, and only able to germinate in that one spot, because there the soil is clear? General Monro, now famous for his unequalled memoir on the bamboos, holds to the latter theory. He pointed out to me that the *Epilobium* seeds, being feathered, could travel with the wind; that the plant always made its appearance first on new banks, landslips, clearings, where it had nothing to compete against; and that the foxglove did the same. True, and most painfully true, in the case of thistles and groundsels: but foxglove seeds, though minute, would hardly be carried by the wind any more than those of the white clover, which comes up so abundantly in drained fens. Adhuc sub judice lis est, and I wish some young naturalists would work carefully at the solution; by experiment, which is the most sure way to find out anything.

But in researches in this direction they will find puzzles enough. I will give them one which I shall be most thankful to hear they have solved within the next seven years—How is it that we find certain plants, namely, the thrift and the scurvy grass, abundant on the sea-shore and common on certain mountain-tops, but nowhere between the two? Answer me that. For I have looked at the fact for years—before, behind, sideways, upside down, and inside out—and I cannot understand it.

But all these questions, and specially, I suspect, that last one, ought to lead the young student up to the great and complex question—How were these islands re-peopled with plants and animals, after the long and wholesale catastrophe of the glacial epoch?

I presume you all know, and will agree, that the whole of these islands, north of the Thames, save certain ice-clad mountain-tops, were buried for long ages under an icy sea. From whence did vegetable and animal life crawl back to the land, as it rose again; and cover its mantle of glacial drift with fresh life and verdure?

Now let me give you a few prolegomena on this matter. You must study the plants of course, species by species. Take Watson's 'Cybele Britannica,' and Moore's 'Cybele Hibernica;' and let—as Mr. Matthew Arnold would say—"your thought play freely about them." Look carefully, too, in the case of each species, at the note on its distribution, which you will find appended in Bentham's 'Handbook,' and in Hooker's 'Student's Flora.' Get all the help you can, if you wish to work the subject out, from foreign botanists, both European and American; and I think that, on the whole, you will come to some such theory as this for a general starting platform. We do not owe our flora—I must keep to the flora just now—to so many different regions, or types, as Mr. Watson conceives, but to three, namely: an European or Germanic flora, from the south-east; an Atlantic flora, from the south-west; a Northern flora from the north. These three invaded us after the glacial epoch; and our general flora is their result.

But this will cause you much trouble. Before you go a step further you will have to eliminate from all your calculations most of the plants which Watson calls glareal, *i.e.* found in cultivated ground about habitations. And what their limit may be I think we never shall know. But of this we may be sure; that just as invading armies always bring with them, in forage or otherwise, some plants from their own country—just as the Cossacks, in 1815, brought more than one Russian plant through Germany into France—just as you have already a crop of North German plants upon the battle-fields of France—thus do conquering races bring new plants. The Romans, during their 300 or 400 years of occupation and civilisation, must have brought more species, I believe, than I dare mention. I suspect them of having brought, not merely the common hedge elm of the south, not merely the three species of nettle, but all our red poppies, and a great number of the weeds which are common in our cornfields; and when we add to them the plants which may have been brought by returning crusaders and pilgrims; by monks from every part of Europe, by Flemings or other dealers in foreign wool; we have to cut a huge cantle out of our indigenous flora: only, having no records, we hardly know where and what to cut out; and can only, we elder ones, recommend the subject to the notice of the younger botanists, that they may work it out after our work is done.

Of course these plants introduced by man, if they are cut out, must be cut out of only one of the floras, namely, the European; for they, probably, came from the south-east, by whatever means they came.

That European flora invaded us, I presume, immediately after the glacial epoch, at a time when France and England were united, and the German Ocean a

mere network of rivers, which emptied into the deep
sea between Scotland and Scandinavia. And here I
must add, that endless questions of interest will arise
to those who will study, not merely the invasion of
that truly European flora, but the invasion of reptiles,
insects, and birds, especially birds of passage, which
must have followed it as soon as the land was sufficiently
covered with vegetation to support life. Whole volumes
remain to be written on this subject. I trust that
some of your younger members may live to write one of
them. The way to begin will be : to compare the flora
and fauna of this part of England very carefully with
that of the southern and eastern counties ; and then to
compare them again with the fauna and flora of France,
Belgium, and Holland.

As for the Atlantic flora, you will have to decide for
yourselves whether you accept or not the theory of a
sunken Atlantic continent. I confess that all objections
to that theory, however astounding it may seem, are
outweighed in my mind by a host of facts which I can
explain by no other theory. But you must judge for
yourselves ; and to do so you must study carefully the
distribution of heaths, both in Europe and at the Cape ;
and their non-appearance beyond the Ural Mountains,
and in America, save in Labrador, where the common
ling, an older and less specialised form, exists. You
must consider, too, the plants common to the Azores,

Portugal, the West of England, Ireland, and the Western Hebrides. In so doing young naturalists will at least find proofs of a change in the distribution of land and water, which will utterly astound them when they face it for the first time.

As for the Northern flora, the question whence it came is puzzling enough. It seems difficult to conceive how any plants could have survived when Scotland was an archipelago in the same ice-covered condition as Greenland is now; and we have no proof that there existed after the glacial epoch any northern continent from which the plants and animals could have come back to us. The species of plants and animals common to Britain, Scandinavia, and North America, must have spread in pre-glacial times, when a continent joining them did exist.

But some light has been thrown on this question by an article, as charming as it is able, on "The Physics of the Arctic Ice," by Dr. Brown, of Campster. You will find it in the 'Quarterly Journal of the Geological Society' for February 1870. He shows there that even in Greenland peaks and crags are left free enough from ice to support a vegetation of between 300 or 400 species of flowering plants; and, therefore, he well says, we must be careful to avoid concluding that the plant and animal life on the dreary shores or mountain-tops of the old glacial Scotland was poor. The same would hold good of our mountains; and, if so, we may look with respect, even with awe, on the Alpine plants of Wales, Scotland, and the Lake mountains, as organisms stunted, it may be, and even degraded, by their long battle with the elements; but venerable from their age, historic from their endurance. Relics of an older temperate world, they have lived through thousands of centuries of frost and fog, to sun themselves in a temperate climate once more. I can never pick one of them without a tinge of shame; and to exterminate one of them is to destroy for the mere pleasure of collecting the last of a family which God has taken the trouble to preserve for thousands of centuries.

I trust that these hints—for I can call them nothing more—will at least awaken any young naturalist who has hitherto only collected natural objects, to study the really important and interesting question—How did these things get here?

Now hence arise questions which may puzzle the mind of a Hampshire naturalist. You have in this neighbourhood, as you well know, two, or rather three, soils, each carrying its peculiar vegetation. First, you have the clay lying on the chalk, and carrying vast woodlands, seemingly primeval. Next, you have the chalk, with its peculiar, delicate, and often fragrant crop of lime-loving plants; and next you have the poor sands and clays of the New Forest basin, saturated with iron, and therefore carrying a moorland or peat-loving vegetation, in many respects quite different from the others. And this moorland soil, and this vegetation, with a few singular exceptions, repeats itself, as I daresay you know, in the north of the county, in the Bagshot basin, as it is called—the moors of Aldershot, Hartford Bridge, and Windsor Forest.

Now what a variety of interesting questions are opened up by these simple facts. How did these three floras get each to its present place? Where did each come from? How did it get past or through the other, till each set of plants, after long internecine competition, settled itself down in the sheet of land most congenial to it? And when did each come hither? Which is the oldest? Will any one tell me whether the healthy floras of the moors, or the thymy flora of the chalk downs, were the earlier inhabitants of these isles? To these questions I cannot get any answer; and they cannot be answered without first—a very careful study of the range of each species of plant on the continent of Europe; and next, without careful study of those stupendous changes in the shape of this island which have taken place at a very late geological epoch. The composition of the flora of our moorlands is as yet to me an utter puzzle. We have Lycopodiums—three species—enormously ancient forms which have survived the age of ice: but did they crawl downward hither from the northern mountains, or upward hither from the Pyrenees? We have the beautiful bog asphodel again—an enormously ancient form; for it is, strange to say, common to North America and to Northern Europe, but does not enter Asia—almost an unique instance. It must, surely, have come from the north; and points—as do many species of plants and animals— to the time when North Europe and North America were joined. We have, sparingly, in North Hampshire, though, strangely, not on the Bagshot moors, the Common or Northern Butterwort (*Pinguicula vulgaris*); and also, in the south, the New Forest part of the county, the delicate little *Pinguicula lusitanica,* the only species now found in Devon and Cornwall, marking the New Forest as the extreme eastern limit of the Atlantic flora. We have again the heaths, which, as I have just said, are found neither in America nor in Asia, and must, I believe, have come from some south-western land long since submerged beneath the sea. But more, we have in the New Forest two plants which are members of the South Europe, or properly, the Atlantic flora; which must have come from the south and south-east; and which are found in no other spots in these islands. I mean the lovely *Gladiolus,* which grows abundantly under the ferns near Lyndhurst, certainly wild, but it does not approach England elsewhere nearer than the Loire and the Rhine; and next, that delicate orchid,

tho *Spiranthes æstivalis*, which is known only in a bog
near Lyndhurst and in the Channel Islands, while on the
Continent it extends from Southern Europe all through
France.   Now, what do these two plants mark ?   They
give us a point in botany, though not in time, to determine when the south of England was parted from
the opposite shores of France ; and whenever that was,
it was just after the Gladiolus and Spiranthes got
hither.   Two little colonies of these lovely flowers
arrived just before their retreat was cut off.   They
found the country already occupied with other plants ;
and, not being reinforced by fresh colonists from the
south, have not been able to spread farther north than
Lyndhurst.   Thus, in the New Forest, and, I may say
in the Bagshot moors, you find plants which you do
not expect, and do not find plants which you do expect ;
and you are, or ought to be, puzzled, and I hope also
interested, and stirred up to find out more.

I spoke just now of the time when England was
joined to France, as bearing on Hampshire botany.   It
bears no less on Hampshire zoology.   In insects, for
instance, the presence of the purple emperor and the
white admiral in our Hampshire woods, as well as
the abundance of the great stag-beetle, point to a time
when the two countries were joined, at least, as far
west as Hampshire ; while the absence of these insects
farther to the westward shows that the countries, if

ever joined, were already parted; and that those insects
have not yet had time to spread westward. The presence of these two butterflies, and partly of the stag-
beetle, along the south-east coast of England as far as
the primeval forests of South Lincolnshire, points—as
do a hundred other facts—to a time when the Straits of
Dover either did not exist, or were the bed of a river
running from the west; and when, as I told you just
now, all the rivers which now run into the German
Ocean, from the Humber on the west to the Elbe on
the east, discharged themselves into the sea between
Scotland and Norway, after wandering through a vast
lowland, covered with countless herds of mammoth,
rhinoceros, gigantic ox, and other mammals now extinct; while the birds, as far as we know; the insects;
the fresh-water fish; and even, as my friend Mr. Brady
has proved, the *Entomostraca* of the rivers, were the
same in what is now Holland as in what is now our
Eastern counties. I could dwell long on this matter.
I could talk long about how certain species of *Lepido-
ptera*—moths and butterflies—like *Papilio Machaon* and
P. Podalirius, swarm through France, reach up to the
British Channel, and have not crossed it; with the
exception of one colony of *Machaon* in the Cambridgeshire fens. I could talk long about a similar phenomenon in the case of our migratory and singing
birds: how many exquisite species—notably those two

glorious songsters, the Orphean Warbler and Hippolais, which delight our ears everywhere on the other side of the Channel—follow our nightingales, blackcaps, and warblers northward every spring almost to the Straits of Dover: but dare not cross, simply because they have been, as it were, created since the gulf was opened, and have never learnt from their parents how to fly over it.

In the case of fishes, again, I might say much on the curious fact that the Cyprinidæ, or white fish—carp, &c.—and their natural enemy, the pike, are indigenous, I believe, only to the rivers, English or continental, on the eastern side of the Straits of Dover; while the rivers on the western side were originally tenanted, like our Hampshire streams, as now, almost entirely by trout, their only Cyprinoid being the minnow—if it, too, be not an interloper; and I might ask you to consider the bearing of this curious fact on the former junction of England and France.

But I have only time to point out to you a few curious facts with regard to reptiles, which should be specially interesting to a Hampshire bio-geologist. You know, of course, that in Ireland there are no reptiles, save the little common lizard, *Lacerta agilis*, and a few frogs on the mountain-tops—how they got there I cannot conceive. And you will, of course, guess, and rightly, that the reason of the absence of reptiles is: that Ireland was parted off from England before the creatures, which certainly spread from southern and warmer climates, had time to get there. You know, of course, that we have a few reptiles in England. But you may not be aware that, as soon as you cross the Channel, you find many more species of reptiles than here, as well as those which you find here. The magnificent green lizard which rattles about like a rabbit in a French forest, is never found here; simply because it had not worked northward till after the Channel was formed. But there are three reptiles peculiar to this part of England which should be most interesting to a Hampshire zoologist. The one is the sand lizard (*L. stirpium*), found on Bourne-heath, and, I suspect, in the South Hampshire moors likewise—a North European and · French species. Another, the *Coronella lævis*, a harmless French and Austrian snake, which has been found about me, in North Hants and South Berks, now about fifteen or twenty times. I have had three specimens from my own parish. I believe it not to be uncommon; and most probably to be found, by those who will look, both in the New Forest and Woolmer. The third is the Natterjack, or running toad (*Bufo Rubeta*), a most beautifully spotted animal, with a yellow stripe down his back, which is common with me at Eversley, and common also in many moorlands of Hants and Surrey;

and, according to Fleming, on heaths near London, and
as far north-east as Lincolnshire; in which case it will
belong to the Germanic fauna.   Now, here again we
have cases of animals which have just been able to get
hither before the severance of England and France;
and which, not being reinforced from the rear, have
been forced to stop, in small and probably decreasing
colonies, on the spots nearest the coast which were fit
for them.

I trust that I have not kept you too long over these
details.   What I wish to impress upon you is that
Hampshire is a country specially fitted for the study of
important bio-geological questions.

To work them out, you must trace the geology of
Hampshire, and, indeed, of East Dorset.   You must try
to form a conception of how the land was shaped in
miocene times, before that tremendous upheaval which
reared the chalk cliffs at Freshwater upright, lifting
the tertiary beds upon their northern slopes.   You
must ask—Was there not land to the south of the Isle
of Wight in those ages, and for ages after; and what
was its extent and shape?   You must ask—When was
the gap between the Isle of Wight and the Isle of Pur-
beck sawn through, leaving the Needles as remnants
on one side, and Old Harry on the opposite?   And was
it sawn asunder merely by the age-long gnawing of
the waves?   You must ask—Where did the great river

which ran from the west, where Poole Harbour is now, and probably through what is now the Solent, depositing brackish water-beds right and left—where, I say, did it run into the sea? Where the Straits of Dover are now? Or, if not there, where? What, too, is become of the land to the Westward, composed of ancient metamorphic rocks, out of which it ran, and deposited on what are now the Haggerstone Moors of Poole, vast beds of grit? What was the climate on its banks when it washed down the delicate leaves of broad-leaved trees, akin to our modern English ones, which are found in the fine mud-sand strata of Bournemouth? When, finally, did it dwindle down to the brook which now runs through Wareham town? Was its bed sea, or dry land, or under an ice sheet, during the long ages of the glacial epoch? And if you say—Who is sufficient for these things?—Who can answer these questions? I answer—Who but you, or your pupils after you, if you will but try?

And if any shall reply—And what use if I do try? What use, if I do try? What use, if I succeed in answering every question which you have propounded to-night? Shall I be the happier for it? Shall I be the wiser?

My friends, whether you will be the happier for it, or for any knowledge of physical science, or for any other knowledge whatsoever, I cannot tell: that lies in the decision of a Higher Power than I; and, indeed, to speak honestly, I do not think that bio-geology or any other branch of physical science is likely, at first at least, to make you happy. Neither is the study of your fellow-men. Neither is religion itself. We were not sent into the world to be happy, but to be right; at least, poor creatures that we are, as right as we can be; and we must be content with being right, and not happy. For I fear, or rather I hope, that most of us are not capable of carrying out Talleyrand's recipe for perfect happiness on earth—namely, a hard heart and a good digestion. Therefore, as our hearts are, happily, not always hard, and our digestions, unhappily, not always good, we will be content to be made wise by physical science, even though we be not made happy.

And we shall be made truly wise if we be made content; content, too, not only with what we can understand, but, content with what we do not understand—the habit of mind which theologians call—and rightly—faith in God; the true and solid faith, which comes often out of sadness, and out of doubt, such as bio-geology may well stir in us at first sight. For our first feeling will be—I know mine was when I began to look into these matters—one somewhat of dread and of horror.

Here were all these creatures, animal and vegetable, competing against each other. And their competition was so earnest and complete, that it did not mean—as

it does among honest shopkeepers in a civilised country
—I will make a little more money than you ; but—I will
crush you, enslave you, exterminate you, eat you up.
"Woe to the weak," seems to be Nature's watchword.
The Psalmist says, "The righteous shall inherit the
land." If you go to a tropical forest, or, indeed, if you
observe carefully a square acre of any English land,
cultivated or uncultivated, you will find that Nature's
text at first sight looks a very different one. She seems
to say—Not the righteous, but the strong, shall inherit
the land. Plant, insect, bird, what not—Find a weaker
plant, insect, bird, than yourself, and kill it, and take
possession of its little vineyard, and no Naboth's curse
shall follow you : but you shall inherit, and thrive
therein, you, and your children after you, if they will
be only as strong and as cruel as you are. That is
Nature's law : and is it not at first sight a fearful law ?
Internecine competition, ruthless selfishness, so internecine and so ruthless that, as I have wandered in tropic
forests, where this temper is shown more quickly and
fiercely, though not in the least more evilly, than in
our slow and cold temperate one, I have said—Really
these trees and plants are as wicked as so many human
beings.

Throughout the great republic of the organic world,
the motto of the majority is, and always has been as far
back as we can see, what it is, and always has been, with

the majority of human beings, "Every one for himself, and the devil take the hindmost." Over-reaching tyranny; the temper which fawns, and clings, and plays the parasite as long as it is down, and when it has risen, fattens on its patron's blood and life—these, and the other works of the flesh, are the works of average plants and animals, as far as they can practise them. At least, so says at first sight the science of bio-geology; till the naturalist, if he be also human and humane, is glad to escape from the confusion and darkness of the universal battle-field of selfishness into the order and light of Christmas-tide.

For then there comes to him the thought—And are these all the facts? And is this all which the facts mean? That mutual competition is one law of Nature, we see too plainly. But is there not, besides that law, a law of mutual help? True it is, as the wise man has said, that the very hyssop on the wall grows there because all the forces of the universe could not prevent its growing. All honour to the hyssop. A brave plant, it has fought a brave fight, and has its just deserts—as everything in Nature has—and so has won. But did all the powers of the universe combine to prevent it growing? Is not that a one-sided statement of facts? Did not all the powers of the universe also combine to make it grow, if only it had valour and worth wherewith to grow? Did not the rains feed it, the very mortar in the wall give lime to its roots? Were not electricity, gravitation, and I know not what of chemical and mechanical forces, busy about the little plant, and every cell of it, kindly and patiently ready to help it, if it would only help itself? Surely this is true; true of every organic thing, animal and vegetable, and mineral, too, for aught I know: and so we must soften our sadness at the sight of the universal mutual war by the sight of an equally universal mutual help.

But more. It is true—too true if you will—that all things live on each other. But is it not, therefore, equally true that all things live for each other?—that self-sacrifice, and not selfishness, is at the bottom the law of Nature, as it is the law of Grace; and the law of bio-geology, as it is the law of all religion and virtue worthy of the name? Is it not true that everything has to help something else to live, whether it knows it or not?—that not a plant or an animal can turn again to its dust without giving food and existence to other plants, other animals?—that the very tiger, seemingly the most useless tyrant of all tyrants, is still of use, when, after sending out of the world suddenly, and all but painlessly, many an animal which would without him have starved in misery through a diseased old age, he himself dies, and, in dying, gives, by his own carcase, the means of life and of enjoyment to a thousandfold more living creatures than ever his paws destroyed?

And so, the longer one watches the great struggle
for existence, the more charitable, the more hopeful,
one becomes; as one sees that, consciously or uncon-
sciously, the law of Nature is, after all, self-sacrifice;
unconscious in plants and animals, as far as we know;
save always those magnificent instances of true self-
sacrifice shown by the social insects, by ants, bees, and
others, which put to shame by a civilization truly noble
—why should I not say divine, for God ordained it?—
the selfishness and barbarism of man.   But be that as
it may, in man the law of self-sacrifice—whether unconscious or not in the animals—rises into consciousness just as far as he is a man; and the crowning
lesson of bio-geology may be, when we have worked it
out, after all, the lesson of Christmas-tide—of the
infinite self-sacrifice of God for man; and Nature as
well as religion may say to us—

> " Ah, could you crush that ever craving lust
> For bliss, which kills all bliss, and lose your life,
> Your barren unit life, to find again
> A thousand times in those for whom you die—
> So were you men and women, and should hold
> Your rightful rank in God's great universe,
> Wherein, in heaven or earth, by will or nature,
> Naught lives for self.   All, all, from crown to base—
> The Lamb, before the world's foundation slain—
> The angels, ministers to God's elect—
> The sun, who only shines to light the worlds—
> The clouds, whose glory is to die in showers—
> The fleeting streams, who in their ocean graves
> Flee the decay of stagnant self-content—

The oak, ennobled by the shipwright's axe—
The soil, which yields its marrow to the flower—
The flower, which feeds a thousand velvet worms
Born only to be prey to every bird—
All spend themselves on others: and shall man,
Whose two-fold being is the mystic knot
Which couples earth with heaven, doubly bound,
As being both worm and angel, to that service
By which both worms and angels hold their life,
Shall he, whose every breath is debt on debt,
Refuse, forsooth, to be what God has made him?
No; let him show himself the creatures' Lord
By free-will gift of that self-sacrifice
Which they, perforce, by Nature's laws endure."

My friends, scientific and others, if the study of bio-geology shall help to teach you this, or anything like this; I think that though it may not make you more happy, it may yet make you more wise; and, therefore, what is better than being more happy, namely, more blessed.

HEROISM.

IT is an open question whether the policeman is not demoralizing us; and that in proportion as he does his duty well; whether the perfection of justice and safety, the complete "preservation of body and goods," may not reduce the educated and comfortable classes into that lap-dog condition in which not conscience, but comfort, doth make cowards of us all. Our forefathers had, on the whole, to take care of themselves; we find it more convenient to hire people to take care of us. So much the better for us, in some respects: but, it may be, so much the worse in others. So much the better; because, as usually results from the division of labour, these people, having little or nothing to do save to take care of us, do so far better than we could; and so prevent a vast amount of violence and wrong, and therefore of misery, especially to the weak: for which last reason we will acquiesce in the existence of police-men and lawyers, as we do in the results of arbitration, as the lesser of two evils. The odds in war are in favour of the bigger bully; in arbitration, in favour of the bigger rogue; and it is a question whether the lion or the fox be the safer guardian of human interests. But arbitration prevents war: and that, in three cases out of four, is full reason for employing it.

On the other hand, the lap-dog condition, whether in dogs or in men, is certainly unfavourable to the growth of the higher virtues. Safety and comfort are good, indeed, for the good; for the brave, the self-originating, the earnest. They give to such a clear stage and no favour wherein to work unhindered for their fellow-men. But for the majority, who are neither brave, self-originating, nor earnest, but the mere puppets of circumstance, safety and comfort may, and actually do, merely make their lives mean and petty, effeminate and dull. Therefore their hearts must be awakened, as often as possible, to take exercise enough for health; and they must be reminded, perpetually and importunately, of what a certain great philosopher called "whatsoever things are true, honourable, just, pure, lovely, and of good report;" "if there be any manhood, and any just praise, to think of such things."

This pettiness and dulness of our modern life is just what keeps alive our stage, to which people go to see something a little less petty, a little less dull, than what they see at home. It is, too, the cause of—I had almost said the excuse for—the modern rage for sensational novels. Those who read them so greedily are conscious, poor souls, of capacities in themselves of passion and action, for good and evil, for which their frivolous humdrum daily life gives no room, no vent. They know too well that human nature can be more fertile, whether in weeds and poisons, or in flowers and fruits, than it is usually in the streets and houses of a well-ordered and tolerably sober city. And because the study of human nature is, after all, that which is nearest to every one and most interesting to every one, therefore they go to fiction, since they cannot go to fact, to see what they themselves might be had they the chance; to see what fantastic tricks before high heaven men and women like themselves can play; and how they play them.

Well: it is not for me to judge, for me to blame. I will only say that there are those who cannot read sensational novels, or, indeed, any novels at all, just because they see so many sensational novels being enacted round them in painful facts of sinful flesh and blood. There are those, too, who have looked in the mirror too often to wish to see their own disfigured visage in it any more; who are too tired of themselves and ashamed of themselves to want to hear of people like themselves; who want to hear of people utterly

unlike themselves, more noble, and able, and just, and
sweet, and pure; who long to hear of heroism and to
converse with heroes; and who, if by chance they meet
with an heroic act, bathe their spirits in that, as in
May-dew, and feel themselves thereby, if but for an
hour, more fair.

If any such shall chance to see these words, let me
ask them to consider with me that one word Hero, and
what it means.

Hero; Heroic; Heroism. These words point to a
phase of human nature, the capacity for which we all
have in ourselves, which is as startling and as interesting in its manifestations as any, and which is always
beautiful, always ennobling, and therefore always at-
tractive to those whose hearts are not yet seared by
the world or brutalized by self-indulgence.

But let us first be sure what the words mean. There
is no use talking about a word till we have got at its
meaning. We may use it as a cant phrase, as a party
cry on platforms; we may even hate and persecute our
fellow-men for the sake of it: but till we have clearly
settled in our own minds what a word means, it will do
for fighting with, but not for working with. Socrates
of old used to tell the young Athenians that the ground
of all sound knowledge was—to understand the true
meaning of the words which were in their mouths all
day long; and Socrates was a wiser man than we shall

ever see. So, instead of beginning an oration in praise of heroism, I shall ask my readers to think with me what heroism is.

Now, we shall always get most surely at the meaning of a word by getting at its etymology—that is, at what it meant at first. And if heroism means behaving like a hero, we must find out, it seems to me, not merely what a hero may happen to mean just now, but what it meant in the earliest human speech in which we find it.

A hero or a heroine, then, among the old Homeric Greeks, meant a man or woman who was like the gods; and who, from that likeness, stood superior to his or her fellow-creatures. Gods, heroes, and men, is a threefold division of rational beings, with which we meet more than once or twice. Those grand old Greeks felt deeply the truth of the poet's saying—

> " Unless above himself he can
> Exalt himself, how poor a thing is man."

But more: the Greeks supposed these heroes to be, in some way or other, partakers of a divine nature; akin to the gods; usually, either they, or some ancestor of theirs, descended from a god or goddess. Those who have read Mr. Gladstone's ' Juventus Mundi' will remember the section (cap. ix. § 6) on the modes of the approximation between the divine and the human natures; and whether or not they agree with the author altogether, all will agree, I think, that the first idea of a hero or a heroine was a godlike man or godlike woman.

A godlike man. What varied, what infinite forms of nobleness that word might include, ever increasing, as men's notions of the gods became purer and loftier, or, alas! decreasing, as their notions became degraded. The old Greeks, with that intense admiration of beauty which made them, in after ages, the master sculptors and draughtsmen of their own, and, indeed, of any age, would, of course, require in their hero, their god-like man, beauty and strength, manners, too, and eloquence, and all outward perfections of humanity, and neglect his moral qualities. Neglect, I say, but not ignore. The hero, by virtue of his kindred with the gods, was always expected to be a better man than common men, as virtue was then understood. And how better? Let us see.

The hero was at least expected to be more reverent than other men to those divine beings of whose nature he partook, whose society he might enjoy even here on earth. He might be unfaithful to his own high lineage; he might misuse his gifts by selfishness and self-will; he might, like Ajax, rage with mere jealousy and wounded pride till his rage ended in shameful madness and suicide. He might rebel against the

very gods, and all laws of right and wrong, till he
perished in his ἀτασθαλίη,

"Smitten down, blind in his pride, for a sign and a terror to mortals."

But he ought to have, he must have, to be true to his
name of Hero, justice, self-restraint, and αἰδώς—that
highest form of modesty, for which we have, alas! no
name in the English tongue; that perfect respect for
the feelings of others which springs out of perfect self-
respect.   And he must have, too—if he were to be a
hero of the highest type—the instinct of helpfulness;
the instinct that, if he were a kinsman of the gods, he
must fight on their side, through toil and danger,
against all that was unlike them, and therefore hateful
to them.   Who loves not the old legends, unsurpassed
for beauty in the literature of any race, in which the
hero stands out as the deliverer, the destroyer of evil?
Theseus ridding the land of robbers, and delivering
it from the yearly tribute of boys and maidens to be
devoured by the Minotaur; Perseus slaying the Gorgon,
and rescuing Andromeda from the sea-beast; Heracles
with his twelve famous labours against giants and
monsters; and all the rest—

> "Who dared, in the god-given might of their manhood
> Greatly to do and to suffer, and far in the fens and the forests
> Smite the devourers of men, heaven-hated, brood of the giants;
> Transformed, strange, without like, who obey not the golden-haired
> rulers"—

These are figures whose divine moral beauty has sunk

into the hearts, not merely of poets or of artists, but of men and women who suffered and who feared; the memory of them, fables though they may have been, ennobled the old Greek heart; they ennobled the heart of Europe in the fifteenth century, at the re-discovery of Greek literature. So far from contradicting the Christian ideal, they harmonised with—I had almost said they supplemented—that more tender and saintly ideal of heroism which had sprung up during the earlier Middle Ages. They justified, and actually gave a new life to, the old noblenesses of chivalry, which had grown up in the later Middle Ages as a necessary supplement of active and manly virtue to the passive and feminine virtue of the cloister. They inspired, mingling with these two other elements, a literature, both in England, France, and Italy, in which the three elements, the saintly, the chivalrous, and the Greek heroic, have become one and undistinguishable, because all three are human, and all three divine; a literature which developed itself in Ariosto, in Tasso, in the Hypnerotomachia, the Arcadia, the Euphues, and other forms, sometimes fantastic, sometimes questionable, but which reached its perfection in our own Spenser's 'Fairy Queen'—perhaps the most admirable poem which has ever been penned by mortal man.

And why? What has made these old Greek myths live, myths though they be, and fables, and fair dreams?

What, though they have no body, and, perhaps, never
had, has given them an immortal soul, which can speak
to the immortal souls of all generations to come?

What but this, that in them—dim it may be and
undeveloped, but still there—lies the divine idea of
self-sacrifice as the perfection of heroism; of self-
sacrifice as the highest duty and the highest joy of
him who claims a kindred with the gods?

Let us say, then, that true heroism must involve
self-sacrifice. Those stories certainly involve it, whether
ancient or modern, which the hearts, not of philosophers
merely, or poets, but of the poorest and the most
ignorant, have accepted instinctively as the highest
form of moral beauty—the highest form, and yet one
possible to all.

Grace Darling rowing out into the storm towards
the wreck.—The "drunken private of the Buffs," who,
prisoner among the Chinese, and commanded to pro-
strate himself and kotoo, refused in the name of his
country's honour—"He would not bow to any China-
man on earth:" and so was knocked on the head, and died
surely a hero's death.—Those soldiers of the 'Birken-
head,' keeping their ranks to let the women and
children escape, while they watched the sharks who in
a few minutes would be tearing them limb from limb.
—Or, to go across the Atlantic—for there are heroes in
the Far West—Mr. Bret Harte's "Flynn of Virginia,"

on the Central Pacific Railway—the place is shown to
travellers—who sacrificed his life for his married com-
rade,—

> " There, in the drift,
> Back to the wall,
> He held the timbers
> Ready to fall.
> Then in the darkness
> I heard him call,—
> ' Run for your life, Jake!
> Run for your wife's sake!
> Don't wait for me.'

> " And that was all
> Heard in the din—
> Heard of Tom Flynn,
> Flynn of Virginia."

Or the engineer, again, on the Mississippi, who, when
the steamer caught fire, held, as he had sworn he would,
her bow against the bank till every soul save he got safe
on shore,—

> " Through the hot black breath of the burning boat
> Jim Bludso's voice was heard ;
> And they all had trust in his cussedness,
> And knew he would keep his word.
> And sure's you're born, they all got off
> Afore the smokestacks fell,—
> And Bludso's ghost went up alone
> In the smoke of the ' Prairie Belle.'

> " He weren't no saint—but at judgment
> I'd run my chance with Jim
> 'Longside of some pious gentlemen
> That wouldn't shake hands with him.
> He'd seen his duty—a dead sure thing—
> And went for it there and then ;
> And Christ is not going to be too hard
> On a man that died for men."

To which gallant poem of Colonel John Hay's—and he
has written many gallant and beautiful poems—I have
but one demurrer: Jim Bludso did not merely do his
duty, but more than his duty. He did a voluntary
deed, to which he was bound by no code or contract,
civil or moral; just as he who introduced me to that
poem won his Victoria Cross—as many a cross, Victoria
and other, has been won—by volunteering for a deed
to which he, too, was bound by no code or contract, military or moral. And it is of the essence of self-sacrifice,
and, therefore, of heroism, that it should be voluntary;
a work of supererogation, at least towards society and
man: an act to which the hero or heroine is not bound
by duty, but which is above though not against duty.

Nay, on the strength of that same element of self-
sacrifice, I will not grudge the epithet heroic, which my
revered friend Mr. Darwin justly applies to the poor
little monkey, who once in his life did that which was
above his duty; who lived in continual terror of the
great baboon, and yet, when the brute had sprung upon
his friend the keeper, and was tearing out his throat,
conquered his fear by love, and, at the risk of instant
death, sprang in turn upon his dreaded enemy, and bit
and shrieked till help arrived.

Some would now-a-days use that story merely to
prove that the monkey's nature and the man's nature
are, after all, one and the same. Well: I, at least,

have never denied that there is a monkey-nature in man, as there is a peacock-nature, and a swine-nature, and a wolf-nature—of all which four I see every day too much. The sharp and stern distinction between men and animals, as far as their natures are concerned, is of a more modern origin than people fancy. Of old the Assyrian took the eagle, the ox, and the lion—and not unwisely—as the three highest types of human capacity. The horses of Homer might be immortal, and weep for their master's death. The animals and monsters of Greek myth—like the Ananzi spider of Negro fable —glide insensibly into speech and reason. Birds —the most wonderful of all animals in the eyes of a man of science or a poet—are sometimes looked on as wiser, and nearer to the gods, than man. The Norseman—the noblest and ablest human being, save the Greek, of whom history can tell us—was not ashamed to say of the bear of his native forests that he had "ten men's strength and eleven men's wisdom." How could Reinecke Fuchs have gained immortality, in the Middle Ages and since, save by the truth of its too solid and humiliating theorem—that the actions of the world of men were, on the whole, guided by passions but too exactly like those of the lower animals? I have said, and say again, with good old Vaughan—

"Unless above himself he can
Exalt himself, how mean a thing is man."

But I cannot forget that many an old Greek poet or sage, and many a sixteenth and seventeenth century one, would have interpreted the monkey's heroism from quite a different point of view; and would have said that the poor little creature had been visited suddenly by some "divine afflatus"—an expression quite as philosophical and quite as intelligible as most philosophic formulas which I read now-a-days—and had been thus raised for the moment above his abject selfish monkey-nature, just as man requires to be raised above his. But that theory belongs to a philosophy which is out of date and out of fashion, and which will have to wait a century or two before it comes into fashion again.

And now: if self-sacrifice and heroism be, as I believe, identical, I must protest against a use of the word sacrifice which is growing too common in newspaper-columns, in which we are told of an "enormous sacrifice of life;" an expression which means merely that a great many poor wretches have been killed, quite against their own will, and for no purpose whatsoever: no sacrifice at all, unless it be one to the demons of ignorance, cupidity or mismanagement.

The stout Whig undergraduate understood better the meaning of such words, who, when asked, "In what sense might Charles the First be said to be a martyr?" answered, "In the same sense that a man might be said to be a martyr to the gout."

And I must protest, in like wise, against a misuse of
the words hero, heroism, heroic, which is becoming too
common, namely, applying them to mere courage. We
have borrowed the misuse, I believe, as we have more
than one beside, from the French press. I trust that
we shall neither accept it, nor the temper which inspires
it. It may be convenient for those who flatter their
nation, and especially the military part of it, into a
ruinous self-conceit, to frame some such syllogism
as this—" Courage is heroism: every Frenchman is
naturally courageous: therefore every Frenchman is a
hero." But we, who have been trained at once in a
sounder school of morals, and in a greater respect for
facts, and for language as the expression of facts, shall
be careful, I hope, not to trifle thus with that potent
and awful engine—human speech. We shall eschew
likewise, I hope, a like abuse of the word moral, which
has crept from the French press now and then, not
only into our own press, but into the writings of some
of our military men, who, as Englishmen, should have
known better. We were told again and again, during
the late war, that the moral effect of such a success had
been great; that the morale of the troops was excellent;
or again, that the morale of the troops had suffered, or
even that they were somewhat demoralised. But when
one came to test what was really meant by these fine
words, one discovered that morals had nothing to do

with the facts which they expressed; that the troops were in the one case actuated simply by the animal passion of hope, in the other simply by the animal passion of fear. This abuse of the word moral has crossed, I am sorry to say, the Atlantic; and a witty American, whom we must excuse, though we must not imitate, when some one had been blazing away at him with a revolver, he being unarmed, is said to have described his very natural emotions on the occasion, by saying that he felt dreadfully demoralised. We, I hope, shall confine the word demoralisation, as our generals of the last century would have done, when applied to soldiers, to crime, including, of course, the neglect of duty or of discipline; and we shall mean by the word heroism in like manner, whether applied to a soldier or to any human being, not mere courage; not the mere doing of duty: but the doing of something beyond duty; something which is not in the bond; some spontaneous and unexpected act of self-devotion.

I am glad, but not surprised, to see that Miss Yonge has held to this sound distinction in her golden little book of 'Golden Deeds;' and said, "Obedience, at all costs and risks, is the very essence of a soldier's life. It has the solid material, but it has hardly the exceptional brightness, of a golden deed."

I know that it is very difficult to draw the line between mere obedience to duty and express heroism.

I know also that it would be both invidious and impertinent in an utterly unheroic personage like me,
to try to draw that line; and to sit at home at ease,
analysing and criticising deeds which I could not do
myself: but—to give an instance or two of what I
mean—

To defend a post as long as it is tenable is not
heroic. It is simple duty. To defend it after it has
become untenable, and even to die in so doing, is not
heroic, but a noble madness, unless an advantage is to
be gained thereby for one's own side. Then, indeed, it
rises towards, if not into, the heroism of self-sacrifice.

Who, for example, will not endorse the verdict of all
ages on the conduct of those Spartans at Thermopylæ,
when they sat "combing their yellow hair for death"
on the sea-shore? They devoted themselves to hopeless destruction: but why? They felt—I must believe
that, for they behaved as if they felt—that on them
the destinies of the Western World might hang; that
they were in the forefront of the battle between civilisation and barbarism, between freedom and despotism;
and that they must teach that vast mob of Persian
slaves, whom the officers of the Great King were
driving with whips up to their lance-points, that the
spirit of the old heroes was not dead; and that the
Greek, even in defeat and death, was a mightier and
a nobler man than they. And they did their work.

They produced, if you will, a "moral" effect, which has lasted even to this very day. They struck terror into the heart, not only of the Persian host, but of the whole Persian empire. They made the event of that war certain, and the victories of Salamis and Platæa comparatively easy. They made Alexander's conquest of the East, 150 years afterwards, not only possible at all, but permanent when it came; and thus helped to determine the future civilisation of the whole world.

They did not, of course, foresee all this. No great or inspired man can foresee all the consequences of his deeds: but these men were, as I hold, inspired to see somewhat at least of the mighty stake for which they played; and to count their lives worthless, if Sparta had sent them thither to help in that great game.

Or shall we refuse the name of heroic to those three German cavalry regiments who, in the battle of Mars La Tour, were bidden to hurl themselves upon the chassepots and mitrailleuses of the unbroken French infantry, and went to almost certain death, over the corpses of their comrades, on and in and through, reeling man over horse, horse over man, and clung like bull-dogs to their work, and would hardly leave, even at the bugle-call, till in one regiment thirteen officers out of nineteen were killed or wounded? And why?

Because the French army must be stopped, if it were but for a quarter of an hour. A respite must be gained for the exhausted Third Corps. And how much might be done, even in a quarter of an hour, by men who knew when, and where, and why to die. Who will refuse the name of heroes to these men? And yet they, probably, would have utterly declined the honour. They had but done that which was in the bond. They were but obeying orders after all. As Miss Yonge well says of all heroic persons—"'I have but done that which it was my duty to do,' is the natural answer of those capable of such actions. They have been constrained to them by duty or pity; have never deemed it possible to act otherwise; and did not once think of themselves in the matter at all."

These last true words bring us to another element in heroism: its simplicity. Whatsoever is not simple; whatsoever is affected, boastful, wilful, covetous, tarnishes, even destroys, the heroic character of a deed; because all these faults spring out of self. On the other hand, wherever you find a perfectly simple, frank, unconscious character, there you have the possibility, at least, of heroic action. For it is nobler far to do the most commonplace duty in the household, or behind the counter, with a single eye to duty, simply because it must be done—nobler far, I say, than to go out of your way to attempt a brilliant deed, with a double mind, and saying to yourself not only—"This will be a brilliant deed," but also—"and it will pay me, or raise me, or set me off, into the bargain." Heroism knows no "into the bargain." And therefore, again, I must protest against applying the word heroic to any deeds, however charitable, however toilsome, however dangerous, performed for the sake of what certain French ladies, I am told, call "faire son salut"—saving one's soul in the world to come. I do not mean to judge. Other and quite unselfish motives may be, and doubtless often are, mixed up with that selfish one : womanly pity and tenderness; love for, and desire to imitate, a certain incarnate ideal of self-sacrifice, who is at once human and divine. But that motive of saving the soul, which is too often openly proposed and proffered, is utterly unheroic. The desire to escape pains and penalties hereafter by pains and penalties here; the balance of present loss against future gain—what is this but selfishness extended out of this world into eternity ? "Not worldliness," indeed, as a satirist once said with bitter truth, "but other-worldliness."

Moreover—and the young and the enthusiastic should also bear this in mind—though heroism means the going beyond the limits of strict duty, it never means the going out of the path of strict duty. If it is your duty to go to London, go thither : you may go as much further as you choose after that. But you must go to London first. Do your duty first; it will be time after that to talk of being heroic.

And therefore one must seriously warn the young, lest they mistake for heroism and self-sacrifice what is merely pride and self-will, discontent with the relations by which God has bound them, and the circumstances which God has appointed for them. I have known girls think they were doing a fine thing by leaving uncongenial parents or disagreeable sisters, and cutting out for themselves, as they fancied, a more useful and elevated line of life than that of mere home duties; while, after all, poor things, they were only saying, with the Pharisees of old, "Corban, it is a gift, by whatsoever thou mightest be profited by me;" and in the name of God, neglecting the command of God to honour their father and mother.

There are men, too, who will neglect their households and leave their children unprovided for, and even uneducated, while they are spending their money on philanthropic or religious hobbies of their own. It is ill to take the children's bread and cast it to the dogs; or even to the angels. It is ill, I say, trying to make God presents, before we have tried to pay God our debts. The first duty of every man is to the wife whom he has married, and to the children whom she has brought into the world; and to neglect them is not heroism, but self-conceit; the conceit that a man is so necessary to Almighty God, that God will actually allow him to do wrong, if He can only thereby secure the man's invaluable services. Be sure that every motive which comes not from the single eye; every motive which springs from self; is by its very essence unheroic, let it look as gaudy or as beneficent as it may.

But I cannot go so far as to say the same of the love of approbation—the desire for the love and respect of our fellow-men.

That must not be excluded from the list of heroic motives. I know that it is, or may be proved to be, by victorious analysis, an emotion common to us and the lower animals. And yet no man excludes it less than that true hero, St. Paul. If those brave Spartans, if those brave Germans, of whom I spoke just now, knew that their memories would be wept over and worshipped by brave men and fair women, and that their names would become watchwords to children in their father-land: what is that to us, save that it should make u? rejoice, if we be truly human, that they had that thought with them in their last moments to make self-devotion more easy, and death more sweet?

And yet—and yet—is not the highest heroism that which is free even from the approbation of our fellow-men, even from the approbation of the best and wisest? The heroism which is known only to our Father who seeth in secret? The Godlike deeds alone in the lonely chamber? The Godlike lives lived in obscurity?—a heroism rare among us men, who live perforce in the glare and noise of the outer world: more common among women; women of whom the world never hears; who, if the world discovered them, would only draw the veil more closely over their faces and their hearts, and entreat to be left alone with God. True, they cannot always hide. They must not always hide; or their fellow-creatures would lose the golden lesson. But, nevertheless, it is of the essence of the perfect and womanly heroism, in which, as in all spiritual forces woman transcends the man, that it would hide if it could.

And it was a pleasant thought to me, when I glanced lately at the golden deeds of woman in Miss Yonge's book—it was a pleasant thought to me, that I could say to myself—Ah! yes. These heroines are known, and their fame flies through the mouths of men. But if so, how many thousands of heroines there must have been, how many thousands there may be now, of whom we shall never know. But still they are there. They sow in secret the seed of which we pluck the flower and eat the fruit, and know not that we pass the sower daily in the street; perhaps some humble, ill-drest woman, earning painfully her own small sustenance. She who nurses a bedridden mother, instead of sending her to the workhouse. She who spends her heart and her money on a drunken father, a reckless brother, on the orphans of a kinsman or a friend. She who — But why go on with the long list of great little heroisms, with which a clergyman at least comes in contact daily —and it is one of the most ennobling privileges of a clergyman's high calling that he does come in contact with them—why go on, I say, save to commemorate one more form of great little heroism—the commonest, and yet the least remembered of all—namely, the heroism of an average mother? Ah, when I think of that last broad fact, I gather hope again for poor humanity; and this dark world looks bright, this diseased world looks wholesome to me once more—because, whatever else it is or is not full of, it is at least full of mothers.

While the satirist only sneers, as at a stock butt for his ridicule, at the managing mother trying to get her daughters married off her hands by chicaneries and meannesses, which every novelist knows too well how to draw—would to heaven he, or rather, alas! she would find some more chivalrous employment for his or her pen—for were they not, too, born of woman?— I only say to myself—having had always a secret fondness for poor Rebecca, though I love Esau more than Jacob—Let the poor thing alone. With pain she brought these girls into the world. With pain she educated them according to her light. With pain she is trying to obtain for them the highest earthly blessing of which she can conceive, namely, to be well married;

and if in doing that last, she manœuvres a little, com-
mits a few basenesses, even tells a few untruths, what
does all that come to, save this—that in the confused
intensity of her motherly self-sacrifice, she will sacrifice
for her daughters even her own conscience and her own
credit? We may sneer, if we will, at such a poor hard-
driven soul when we meet her in society: our duty, both
as Christians and ladies and gentlemen, seems to me to
be—to do for her something very different indeed.

But to return. Looking at the amount of great
little heroisms, which are being, as I assert, enacted
around us every day, no one has a right to say, what
we are all tempted to say at times—"How can I be
heroic? This is no heroic age, setting me heroic
examples. We are growing more and more comfortable,
frivolous, pleasure-seeking, money-making; more and
more utilitarian; more and more mercenary in our
politics, in our morals, in our religion; thinking less
and less of honour and duty, and more and more of loss
and gain. I am born into an unheroic time. You
must not ask me to become heroic in it."

I do not deny that it is more difficult to be heroic,
while circumstances are unheroic round us. We are
all too apt to be the puppets of circumstances; all too
apt to follow the fashion; all too apt, like so many
minnows, to take our colour from the ground on which
we lie, in hopes, like them, of comfortable concealment,

lest the new tyrant deity, called public opinion, should spy us out, and, like Nebuchadnezzar of old, cast us into a burning fiery furnace—which public opinion can make very hot—for daring to worship any god or man save the will of the temporary majority.

Yes, it is difficult to be anything but poor, mean, insufficient, imperfect people, as like each other as so many sheep; and, like so many sheep, having no will or character of our own, but rushing altogether blindly over the same gap, in foolish fear of the same dog, who, after all, dare not bite us; and so it always was and always will be.

For the third time I say,—

> "Unless above himself he can
> Exalt himself, how poor a thing is man."

But, nevertheless, any man or woman who will, in any age and under any circumstances, can live the heroic life and exercise heroic influences.

If any ask proof of this, I shall ask them, in return, to read two novels; novels, indeed, but, in their method and their moral, partaking of that heroic and ideal element, which will make them live, I trust, long after thousands of mere novels have returned to their native dust. I mean Miss Muloch's 'John Halifax, Gentleman,' and Mr. Thackeray's 'Esmond,' two books which no man or woman ought to read without being the nobler for them.

'John Halifax, Gentleman,' is simply the history of a poor young clerk, who rises to be a wealthy mill-owner in the manufacturing districts, in the early part of this century. But he contrives to be an heroic and ideal clerk, and an heroic and ideal mill-owner; and that without doing anything which the world would call heroic or ideal, or in anywise stepping out of his sphere, minding simply his own business, and doing the duty which lies nearest him. And how? By getting into his head from youth the strangest notion, that in whatever station or business he may be, he can always be what he considers a gentleman; and that if he only behaves like a gentleman, all must go right at last. A beautiful book. As I said before, somewhat of an heroic and ideal book. A book which did me good when first I read it; which ought to do any young man good who will read it, and then try to be, like John Halifax, a gentleman, whether in the shop, the counting-house, the bank, or the manufactory.

The other—an even more striking instance of the possibility, at least, of heroism anywhere and everywhere—is Mr. Thackeray's 'Esmond.' On the meaning of that book I can speak with authority. For my dear and regretted friend told me himself that my interpretation of it was the true one; that this was the lesson which he meant men to learn therefrom.

Esmond is a man of the first half of the eighteenth

Q

century; living in a coarse, drunken, ignorant, profligate, and altogether unheroic age. He is—and here the high art and the high morality of Mr. Thackeray's genius is shown—altogether a man of his own age. He is not a sixteenth-century or a nineteenth-century man born out of time. His information, his politics, his religion, are no higher than of those round him. His manners, his views of human life, his very prejudices and faults, are those of his age. The temptations which he conquers are just those under which the men around him fall. But how does he conquer them? By holding fast throughout to honour, duty, virtue. Thus, and thus alone, he becomes an ideal eighteenth-century gentleman, an eighteenth-century hero. This was what Mr. Thackeray meant—for he told me so himself, I say—that it was possible, even in England's lowest and foulest times, to be a gentleman and a hero, if a man would but be true to the light within him.

But I will go further. I will go from ideal fiction to actual, and yet ideal, fact; and say that, as I read history, the most unheroic age which the civilized world ever saw was also the most heroic; that the spirit of man triumphed most utterly over his circumstances, at the very moment when those circumstances were most against him.

How and why he did so is a question for philosophy in the highest sense of that word. The fact of his having done so is matter of history. Shall I solve my own riddle?

Then, have we not heard of the early Christian martyrs? Is there a doubt that they, unlettered men, slaves, weak women, even children, did exhibit, under an infinite sense of duty, issuing in infinite self-sacrifice, a heroism such as the world had never seen before; did raise the ideal of human nobleness a whole stage—rather say, a whole heaven—higher than before; and that wherever the tale of their great deeds spread, men accepted, even if they did not copy, those martyrs as ideal specimens of the human race, till they were actually worshipped by succeeding generations, wrongly, it may be, but pardonably, as a choir of lesser deities?

But is there, on the other hand, a doubt that the age in which they were heroic was the most unheroic of all ages; that they were bred, lived, and died, under the most debasing of materialist tyrannies, with art, literature, philosophy, family and national life dying or dead around them, and in cities the corruption of which cannot be told for very shame—cities, compared with which Paris is the abode of Arcadian simplicity and innocence? When I read Petronius and Juvenal, and recollect that they were the contemporaries of the Apostles; when — to give an instance which scholars, and perhaps, happily, only scholars, can appreciate—I glance once more at Trimalchio's feast.

and remember that within a mile of that feast St. Paul may have been preaching to a Christian congregation, some of whom—for St. Paul makes no secret of that strange fact—may have been, ere their conversion, partakers in just such vulgar and bestial orgies as those which were going on in the rich freedman's halls: after that, I say, I can put no limit to the possibility of man's becoming heroic, even though he be surrounded by a hell on earth; no limit to the capacities of any human being to form for himself or herself a high and pure ideal of human character; and, without "playing fantastic tricks before high heaven," to carry out that ideal in every-day life; and in the most commonplace circumstances, and the most menial occupations, to live worthy of—as I conceive—our heavenly birthright, and to imitate the heroes, who were the kinsmen of the gods.

SUPERSTITION.

A LECTURE DELIVERED AT THE ROYAL INSTITUTION, LONDON.

———◦◦◦———

HAVING accepted the very great honour of being allowed to deliver here two lectures, I have chosen as my subject Superstition and Science. It is with Superstition that this first lecture will deal.

The subject seems to me especially fit for a clergyman; for he should, more than other men, be able to avoid trenching on two subjects rightly excluded from this Institution; namely, Theology—that is, the knowledge of God; and Religion—that is, the knowledge of Duty. If he knows, as he should, what is Theology, and what is Religion, then he should best know what is not Theology, and what is not Religion.

For my own part, I entreat you at the outset to keep in mind that these lectures treat of matters entirely physical; which have in reality, and ought to have in our minds, no more to do with Theology and Religion than the proposition that theft is wrong, has to do with the proposition that the three angles of a triangle are equal to two right angles.

It is necessary to premise this, because many are of opinion that superstition is a corruption of religion; and though they would agree that as such, "corruptio optimi pessima," yet they would look on religion as the state of spiritual health, and superstition as one of spiritual disease.

Others, again, holding the same notion, but not considering that corruptio optimi pessima, have been in all ages somewhat inclined to be merciful to superstition, as a child of reverence; as a mere accidental misdirection of one of the noblest and most wholesome faculties of man.

This is not the place wherein to argue with either of these parties; and I shall simply say that superstition seems to me altogether a physical affection, as thoroughly material and corporeal as those of eating or sleeping, remembering or dreaming.

After this, it will be necessary to define superstition, in order to have some tolerably clear understanding of what we are talking about. I beg leave to define it as —Fear of the unknown.

Johnson, who was no dialectician, and, moreover, superstitious enough himself, gives eight different definitions of the word; which is equivalent to confessing his inability to define it at all :—

" 1. Unnecessary fear or scruples in religion; observance of unnecessary and uncommanded rites or practices; religion without morality.

" 2. False religion; reverence of beings not proper objects of reverence; false worship.

" 3. Over nicety; exactness too scrupulous."

Eight meanings; which, on the principle that eight eighths, or indeed 800, do not make one whole, may be considered as no definition. His first thought, as often happens, is the best—"Unnecessary fear." But after that he wanders. The root-meaning of the word is still to seek. But, indeed, the popular meaning, thanks to popular common sense, will generally be found to contain in itself the root-meaning.

Let us go back to the Latin word Superstitio. Cicero says that the superstitious element consists in " a certain empty dread of the gods "—a purely physical affection, if you will remember three things :—

1. That dread is in itself a physical affection.

2. That the gods who were dreaded were, with the vulgar, who alone dreaded them, merely impersonations of the powers of nature.

3. That it was physical injury which these gods were expected to inflict.

But he himself agrees with this theory of mine; for he says shortly after, that not only philosophers, but even the ancient Romans, had separated superstition from

religion; and that the word was first applied to those
who prayed all day ut liberi sui sibi superstites essent
—might survive them.   On the etymology no one will
depend who knows the remarkable absence of any
etymological instinct in the ancients, in consequence of
their weak grasp of that sound inductive method which
has created modern criticism.   But if it be correct, it
is a natural and pathetic form for superstition to take
in the minds of men who saw their children fade and
die ;   probably the greater number of them beneath
diseases which mankind could neither comprehend nor
cure.

The best exemplification of what the ancients meant
by superstition is to be found in the lively and dramatic
words of Aristotle's great pupil, Theophrastus.

The superstitious man, according to him, after having
washed his hands with lustral water—that is, water in
which a torch from the altar had been quenched, goes
about with a laurel-leaf in his mouth, to keep off evil
influences, as the pigs in Devonshire used, in my youth,
to go about with a withe of mountain ash round their
necks to keep off the evil eye.   If a weasel crosses his
path, he stops, and either throws three pebbles into
the road, or, with the innate selfishness of fear, lets
some one else go before him, and attract to himself the
harm which may ensue.   He has a similar dread of a
screech-owl, whom he compliments in the name of its

mistress, Pallas Athene. If he finds a serpent in his
house, he sets up an altar to it. If he pass at a four-
cross-way an anointed stone, he pours oil on it, kneels
down, and adores it. If a rat has nibbled one of his
sacks he takes it for a fearful portent—a superstition
which Cicero also mentions. He dare not sit on a
tomb, because it would be assisting at his own funeral.
He purifies endlessly his house, saying that Hecate—
that is, the moon—has exercised some malign influence
on it; and many other purifications he observes, of
which I shall only say that they are by their nature
plainly, like the last, meant as preservatives against
unseen malarias or contagions, possible or impossible.
He assists every month with his children at the
mysteries of the Orphic priests; and finally, whenever
he sees an epileptic patient, he spits in his own bosom
to avert the evil omen.

I have quoted, I believe, every fact given by Theophrastus; and you will agree, I am sure, that the
moving and inspiring element of such a character is
mere bodily fear of unknown evil. The only superstition attributed to him which does not at first sight
seem to have its root in dread is that of the Orphic
mysteries. But of them Müller says that the Dionusos
whom they worshipped " was an infernal deity, connected with Hades, and was the personification, not
merely of rapturous pleasure, but of a deep sorrow for

the miseries of human life." The Orphic societies of Greece seem to have been peculiarly ascetic, taking no animal food save raw flesh from the sacrificed ox of Dionusos. And Plato speaks of a lower grade of Orphic priests, Orpheotelestai, "who used to come before the doors of the rich, and promise, by sacrifices and expiatory songs, to release them from their own sins, and those of their forefathers;" and such would be but too likely to get a hearing from the man who was afraid of a weasel or an owl.

Now, this same bodily fear, I verily believe, will be found at the root of all superstition whatsoever.

But be it so. Fear is a natural passion, and a wholesome one. Without the instinct of self-preservation, which causes the sea-anemone to contract its tentacles, or the fish to dash into its hover, species would be extermined wholesale by involuntary suicide.

Yes; fear is wholesome enough, like all other faculties, as long as it is controlled by reason. But what if the fear be not rational, but irrational? What if it be, in plain homely English, blind fear; fear of the unknown, simply because it is unknown? Is it not likely, then, to be afraid of the wrong object? to be hurtful, ruinous to animals as well as to man? Any one will confess that, who has ever seen a horse inflict on himself mortal injuries, in his frantic attempts to escape from a quite imaginary danger. I have good reasons for believing

that not only animals here and there, but whole flocks
and swarms of them, are often destroyed, even in the
wild state, by mistaken fear ; by such panics, for
instance, as cause a whole herd of buffalos to rush over
a bluff, and be dashed to pieces. And remark that this
capacity of panic, fear—of superstition, as I should call
it—is greatest in those animals, the dog and the horse
for instance, which have the most rapid and vivid fancy.
Does not the unlettered Highlander say all that I want
to say, when he attributes to his dog and his horse, on
the strength of these very manifestations of fear, the
capacity of seeing ghosts and fairies before he can see
them himself ?

But blind fear not only causes evil to the coward
himself : it makes him a source of evil to others ; for it
is the cruellest of all human states.   It transforms the
man into the likeness of the cat, who, when she is
caught in a trap, or shut up in a room, has too low an
intellect to understand that you wish to release her ;
and, in the madness of terror, bites and tears at the
hand which tries to do her good.   Yes ; very cruel is
blind fear.   When a man dreads he knows not what, he
will do he cares not what.   When he dreads desperately,
he will act desperately.   When he dreads beyond all
reason, he will behave beyond all reason.   He has no
law of guidance left, save the lowest selfishness.   No
law of guidance : and yet his intellect, left unguided,

may be rapid and acute enough to lead him into terrible follies. Infinitely more imaginative than the lowest animals, he is for that very reason capable of being infinitely more foolish, more cowardly, more superstitious. He can—what the lower animals, happily for them, cannot—organise his folly; erect his superstitions into a science; and create a whole mythology out of his blind fear of the unknown. And when he has done that—Woe to the weak! For when he has reduced his superstition to a science, then he will reduce his cruelty to a science likewise, and write books like the Malleus Maleficarum, and the rest of the witch-literature of the fifteenth, sixteenth, and seventeenth centuries; of which Mr. Lecky has of late told the world so much, and told it most faithfully and most fairly.

But, fear of the unknown? Is not that fear of the unseen world? And is not that fear of the spiritual world? Pardon me: a great deal of that fear—all of it, indeed, which is superstition—is simply not fear of the spiritual, but of the material; and of nothing else.

The spiritual world—I beg you to fix this in your minds—is not merely an invisible world which may become visible, but an invisible world which is by its essence invisible; a moral world, a world of right and wrong. And spiritual fear—which is one of the noblest of all affections, as bodily fear is one of the basest—is, if properly defined, nothing less or more than the fear of doing wrong; of becoming a worse man.

But what has that to do with mere fear of the unseen? The fancy which conceives the fear is physical, not spiritual. Think for yourselves. What difference is there between a savage's fear of a demon, and a hunter's fear of a fall? The hunter sees a fence. He does not know what is on the other side: but he has seen fences like it with a great ditch on the other side, and suspects one here likewise. He has seen horses fall at such, and men hurt thereby. He pictures to himself his horse falling at that fence, himself rolling in the ditch, with possibly a broken limb; and he recoils from the picture he himself has made; and perhaps with very good reason. His picture may have its counterpart in fact; and he may break his leg. But his picture, like the previous pictures from which it was compounded, is simply a physical impression on the brain, just as much as those in dreams.

Now, does the fact of the ditch, the fall, and the broken leg, being unseen and unknown, make them a spiritual ditch, a spiritual fall, a spiritual broken leg? And does the fact of the demon and his doings, being as yet unseen and unknown, make them spiritual, or the harm that he may do, a spiritual harm? What does the savage fear? Lest the demon should appear; that is, become obvious to his physical senses, and produce an unpleasant physical effect on them. He fears lest the fiend should entice him into the bog, break the hand-bridge over the brook, turn into a horse and ride away with him, or jump out from behind a tree and wring his neck—tolerably hard physical facts, all of them; the children of physical fancy, regarded with physical dread. Even if the superstition proved true; even if the demon did appear; even if he wrung the traveller's neck in sound earnest, there would be no more spiritual agency or phenomenon in the whole tragedy than there is in the parlour table, when spiritual somethings make spiritual raps upon spiritual wood; and human beings, who are really spirits—and would to heaven they would remember that fact, and what it means—believe that anything has happened beyond a clumsy juggler's trick.

You demur? Do you not see that the demon, by the mere fact of having produced physical consequences, would have become himself a physical agent, a member of physical Nature, and therefore to be explained, he and his doings, by physical laws? If you do not see that conclusion at first sight, think over it till you do.

It may seem to some that I have founded my theory on a very narrow basis; that I am building up an inverted pyramid; or that, considering the numberless, complex, fantastic shapes which superstition has assumed, bodily fear is too simple to explain them all.

But if those persons will think a second time, they must agree that my base is as broad as the phenomena which it explains; for every man is capable of fear. And they will see, too, that the cause of superstition must be something like fear, which is common to all men : for all, at least as children, are capable of superstition; and that it must be something which, like fear, is of a most simple, rudimentary, barbaric kind; for the lowest savage, of whatever he is not capable, is still superstitious, often to a very ugly degree. Superstition seems, indeed, to be, next to the making of stone-weapons, the earliest method of asserting his superiority to the brutes which has occurred to that utterly abnormal and fantastic lusus naturæ called man.

Now let us put ourselves awhile, as far as we can, in the place of that same savage ; and try whether my theory will not justify itself; whether or not superstition, with all its vagaries, may have been, indeed must have been, the result of that ignorance and fear which he carried about with him, every time he prowled for food through the primeval forest.

A savage's first division of nature would be, I should say, into things which he can eat and things which can eat him ; including, of course, his most formidable enemy, and most savoury food—his fellow-man. In finding out what he can eat, we must remember, he will have gone through much experience which will have inspired him with a serious respect for the hidden wrath of nature; like those Himalayan folk, of whom Hooker says, that as they know every poisonous plant, they must have tried them all—not always with impunity.

So he gets at a third class of objects—things which he cannot eat, and which will not eat him; but will only do him harm, as it seems to him, out of pure malice, like poisonous plants and serpents. There are natural accidents, too, which fall into the same category, stones, floods, fires, avalanches. They hurt him or kill him, surely for ends of their own. If a rock falls from the cliff above him, what more natural than to suppose that there is some giant up there who threw it at him? If he had been up there, and strong enough, and had seen a man walking underneath, he would certainly have thrown the stone at him and killed him. For first, he might have eaten the man after; and even if he were not hungry, the man might have done him a mischief; and it was prudent to prevent that, by doing him a mischief first. Besides, the man might have a wife; and if he killed the man, then the wife would, by a very ancient law common to man and animals, become the prize of the victor. Such is the natural man, the carnal man, the soulish man, the ἄνθρωπος ψυχικὸς of St. Paul, with five tolerably acute senses, which are ruled by five very acute animal passions—

hunger, sex, rage, vanity, fear. It is with the working of the last passion, fear, that this lecture has to do.

So the savage concludes that there must be a giant living in the cliff, who threw stones at him, with evil intent; and he concludes in like wise concerning most other natural phenomena. There is something in them which will hurt him, and therefore likes to hurt him : and if he cannot destroy them, and so deliver himself, his fear of them grows quite boundless. There are hundreds of natural objects on which he learns to look with the same eyes as the little boys of Teneriffe look on the useless and poisonous *Euphorbia canariensis.* It is to them—according to Mr. Piazzi Smyth—a demon who would kill them, if it could only run after them ; but as it cannot, they shout Spanish curses at it, and pelt it with volleys of stones, "screeching with elfin joy, and using worse names than ever, when the poisonous milk spurts out from its bruised stalks."

And if such be the attitude of the uneducated man towards the permanent terrors of nature, what will it be towards those which are sudden and seemingly capricious?—towards storms, earthquakes, floods, blights, pestilences? We know too well what it has been—one of blind, and therefore often cruel, fear. How could it be otherwise? . Was Theophrastus's superstitious man so very foolish for pouring oil on every round stone? I think there was a great deal to be said for him. . This

R

worship of Bætyli was rational enough. They were
acrolites, fallen from heaven. Was it not as well to be
civil to such messengers from above?—to testify by
homage to them due awe of the being who had thrown
them at men, and who though he had missed his shot
that time, might not miss it the next? I think if we,
knowing nothing of either gunpowder, astronomy, or
Christianity, saw an Armstrong bolt fall within five
miles of London, we should be inclined to be very
respectful to it indeed. So the acrolites, or glacial
boulders, or polished stone weapons of an extinct
race, which looked like acrolites, were the children of
Ouranos the heaven, and had souls in them. One,
by one of those strange transformations in which the
logic of unreason indulges, the image of Diana of the
Ephesians, which fell down from Jupiter; another was
the Ancile, the holy shield which fell from the same
place in the days of Numa Pompilius, and was the
guardian genius of Rome; and several more became
notable for ages.

Why not? The uneducated man of genius, un-
acquainted alike with metaphysics and with biology,
sees, like a child, a personality in every strange and
sharply-defined object. A cloud like an angel may
be an angel; a bit of crooked root like a man may be a
man turned into wood—perhaps to be turned back again
at its own will. An erratic block has arrived where it

is by strange unknown means. Is not that an evidence
of its personality? Either it has flown hither itself, or
some one has thrown it. In the former case, it has life,
and is proportionally formidable; in the latter, he who
had thrown it is formidable.

I know two erratic blocks of porphyry—I believe there
are three—in Cornwall, lying one on serpentine, one,
I think, on slate, which—so I was always informed as a
boy—were the stones which St. Kevern threw after St.
Just when the latter stole his host's chalice and paten,
and ran away with them to the Land's End. Why
not? Before we knew anything about the action of
icebergs and glaciers, that is, until the last eighty years,
that was as good a story as any other; while how life-
like these boulders are, let a great poet testify; for the
fact has not escaped the delicate eye of Wordsworth:

> " As a huge stone is sometimes seen to lie
> Couched on the bald top of an eminence;
> Wonder to all who do the same espy,
> By what means it could thither come, and whence,
> So that it seems a thing endued with sense;
> Like a sea-beast crawled forth, that on a shelf
> Of rock or sand reposeth, there to sun itself."

To the civilised poet, the fancy becomes a beautiful
simile; to a savage poet, it would have become a material
and a very formidable fact. He stands in the
valley, and looks up at the boulder on the far-off fells.
He is puzzled by it. He fears it. At last he makes up

his mind. It is alive. As the shadows move over it, he sees it move. May it not sleep there all day, and prowl for prey all night? He had been always afraid of going up those fells; now he will never go. There is a monster there.

Childish enough, no doubt. But remember that the savage is always a child. So, indeed, are millions, as well clothed, housed, and policed as ourselves—children from the cradle to the grave. But of them I do not talk; because, happily for the world, their childishness is so overlaid by the result of other men's manhood; by an atmosphere of civilisation and Christianity which they have accepted at second-hand as the conclusions of minds wiser than their own, that they do all manner of reasonable things for bad reasons, or for no reason at all, save the passion of imitation. Not in them, but in the savage, can we see man as he is by nature, the puppet of his senses and his passions, the natural slave of his own fears.

But has the savage no other faculties, save his five senses and five passions? I do not say that. I should be most unphilosophical if I said it; for the history of mankind proves that he has infinitely more in him than that. Yes: but in him that infinite more, which is not only the noblest part of humanity, but, it may be, humanity itself, is not to be counted as one of the roots of superstition. For in the savage man, in whom superstition certainly originates, that infinite more is still merely in him; inside him; a faculty: but not yet a fact.   It has not come out of him into consciousness, purpose, and act; and is to be treated as non-existent: while what has come out, his passions and senses, is enough to explain all the vagaries of superstition; a vera causa for all its phenomena.   And if we seem to have found a sufficient explanation already, it is un-philosophical to look further, at least till we have tried whether our explanation fits the facts.

Nevertheless, there is another faculty in the savage, to which I have already alluded, common to him and to at least the higher vertebrates—fancy; the power of reproducing internal images of external objects, whether in its waking form of physical memory—if, indeed, all memory be not physical—or in its sleeping form of dreaming.   Upon this last, which has played so very important a part in superstition in all ages, I beg you to think a moment.   Recollect your own dreams during childhood; and recollect again that the savage is always a child.   Recollect how difficult it was for you in childhood, how difficult it must be always for the savage, to decide whether dreams are phantasms or realities.   To the savage, I doubt not, the food he eats, the foes he grapples with, in dreams, are as real as any waking impressions.   But, moreover, these dreams will be very often, as children's dreams are wont to be, of a painful and terrible kind. Perhaps they will be always painful; perhaps his dull brain will never dream, save under the influence of indigestion, or hunger, or an uncomfortable attitude. And so, in addition to his waking experience of the terrors of nature, he will have a whole dream-experience besides, of a still more terrific kind. He walks by day past a black cavern mouth, and thinks, with a shudder—Something ugly may live in that ugly hole : what if it jumped out upon me? He broods over the thought with the intensity of a narrow and unoccupied mind; and a few nights after, he has eaten—but let us draw a veil before the larder of a savage—his chin is pinned down on his chest, a slight congestion of the brain comes on; and behold he finds himself again at that cavern's mouth, and something ugly does jump out upon him : and the cavern is a haunted spot henceforth to him and to all his tribe. It is in vain that his family tell him that he has been lying asleep at home all the while. He has the evidence of his senses to prove the contrary. He must have got out of himself, and gone into the woods. When we remember that certain wise Greek philosophers could find no better explanation of dreaming than that the soul left the body, and wandered free, we cannot condemn the savage for his theory.

Now, I submit that in these simple facts we have a

group of "true causes" which are the roots of all the
superstitions of the world.

And if any one shall complain that I am talking
materialism: I shall answer, that I am doing exactly
the opposite. I am trying to eliminate and get rid of
that which is material, animal, and base; in order that
that which is truly spiritual may stand out, distinct
and clear, in its divine and eternal beauty.

To explain, and at the same time, as I think, to
verify my hypothesis, let me give you an example—
fictitious, it is true, but probable fact nevertheless;
because it is patched up of many fragments of actual
fact: and let us see how, in following it out, we shall
pass through almost every possible form of superstition.

Suppose a great hollow tree, in which the formidable
wasps of the tropics have built for ages. The average
savage hurries past the spot in mere bodily fear; for
if they come out against him, they will sting him to
death; till at last there comes by a savage wiser than
the rest, with more observation, reflection, imagination,
independence of will—the genius of his tribe.

The awful shade of the great tree, added to his terror
of the wasps, weighs on him, and excites his brain.
Perhaps, too, he has had a wife or a child stung to
death by these same wasps. These wasps, so small,
yet so wise, far wiser than he: they fly, and they

sting. Ah, if he could fly and sting; how he would kill and eat, and live right merrily. They build great towns; they rob far and wide; they never quarrel with each other: they must have some one to teach them, to lead them—they must have a king. And so he gets the fancy of a Wasp-King; as the western Irish still believe in the Master Otter; as the Red Men believe in the King of the Buffalos, and find the bones of his ancestors in the Mammoth remains of Big-bone Lick; as the Philistines of Ekron—to quote a notorious instance—actually worshipped Baal-zebub, lord of the flies.

If they have a king, he must be inside that tree, of course. If he, the savage, were a king, he would not work for his bread, but sit at home and make others feed him; and so, no doubt, does the wasp-king.

And when he goes home he will brood over this wonderful discovery of the wasp-king; till, like a child, he can think of nothing else. He will go to the tree, and watch for him to come out. The wasps will get accustomed to his motionless figure, and leave him unhurt; till the new fancy will rise in his mind that he is a favourite of this wasp-king: and at last he will find himself grovelling before the tree, saying—"Oh great wasp-king, pity me, and tell your children not to sting me, and I will bring you honey, and fruit, and flowers to eat, and I will flatter you, and worship you, and you shall be my king."

And then he would gradually boast of his discovery; of the new mysterious bond between him and the wasp-king; and his tribe would believe him, and fear him; and fear him still more when he began to say, as he surely would, not merely—"I can ask the wasp-king, and he will tell his children not to sting you:" but— "I can ask the wasp-king, and he will send his children, and sting you all to death." Vanity and ambition will have prompted the threat: but it will not be altogether a lie. The man will more than half believe his own words; he will quite believe them when he has repeated them a dozen times.

And so he will become a great man, and a king, under the protection of the king of the wasps; and he will become, and it may be his children after him, priest of the wasp-king, who will be their fetish, and the fetish of their tribe.

And they will prosper, under the protection of the wasp-king. The wasp will become their moral ideal, whose virtues they must copy. The new chief will preach to them wild eloquent words. They must sting like wasps, revenge like wasps, hold all together like wasps, build like wasps, work hard like wasps, rob like wasps; then, like the wasps, they will be the terror of all around, and kill and eat all their enemies. Soon

they will call themselves The Wasps. They will boast
that their king's father or grandfather, and soon thr.'
the ancestor of the whole tribe, was an actual wasp;
and the wasp will become at once their eponym hero,
their deity, their ideal, their civiliser; who has taught
them to build a kraal of huts, as he taught his children
to build a hive.

Now, if there should come to any thinking man of
this tribe, at this epoch, the new thought—Who made
the world? he will be sorely puzzled. The conception
of a world has never crossed his mind before. He never
pictured to himself anything beyond the nearest ridge
of mountains; and as for a Maker, that will be a greater
puzzle still. What makers or builders more cunning
than those wasps of whom his foolish head is full? Of
course, he sees it now. A Wasp made the world; which ·
to him entirely new guess might become an integral
part of his tribe's creed. That would be their cos-
mogony. And if, a generation or two after, another
savage genius should guess that the world was a globe
hanging in the heavens, he would, if he had imagination
enough to take the thought in at all, put it to himself
in a form suited to his previous knowledge and conceptions. It would seem to him that The Wasp flew about
the skies with the world in his mouth, as he carries a
bluebottle fly; and that would be the astronomy of his
tribe henceforth. Absurd enough; but—as every man :

who is acquainted with old mythical cosmogonies must
know—no more absurd than twenty similar guesses on
record. Try to imagine the gradual genesis of such
myths as the Egyptian scarabæus and egg, or the Hindoo
theory that the world stood on an elephant, the elephant
on a tortoise, the tortoise on that infinite note of in-
terrogation which, as some one expresses it, underlies all
physical speculations, and judge: must they not have
arisen in some such fashion as that which I have
pointed out?

This, I say, would be the culminating point of the
wasp-worship, which had sprung up out of bodily fear
of being stung.

But times might come for it in which it would go
through various changes, through which every superstition in the world, I suppose, has passed or is doomed
to pass.

The wasp-men might be conquered, and possibly
eaten, by a stronger tribe than themselves. What
would be the result? They would fight valiantly at
first, like wasps. But what if they began to fail?
Was not the wasp-king angry with them? Had not he
deserted them? He must be appeased; he must have
his revenge. They would take a captive, and offer him
to the wasps. So did a North American tribe, in their
need, some forty years ago; when, because their maize-
crops failed, they roasted alive a captive girl, cut her

to pieces, and sowed her with their corn. I would not
tell the story, for the horror of it, did it not bear with
such fearful force on my argument. What were those
Red Men thinking of? What chain of misreasoning
had they in their heads when they hit on that as a
device for making the crops grow? Who can tell?
Who can make the crooked straight, or number that
which is wanting? As said Solomon of old, so must
we—" The foolishness of fools is folly." One thing
only we can say of them, that they were horribly afraid
of famine, and took that means of ridding themselves of
their fear.

But what if the wasp tribe had no captives? They
would offer slaves. What if the agony and death of
slaves did not appease the wasps? They would offer
their fairest, their dearest, their sons and their
daughters, to the wasps; as the Carthaginians, in like
strait, offered in one day 200 noble boys to Moloch, the
volcano-god, whose worship they had brought out of
Syria; whose original meaning they had probably forgotten; of whom they only knew that he was a dark
and devouring being, who must be appeased with the
burning bodies of their sons and daughters. And so
the veil of fancy would be lifted again, and the whole
superstition stand forth revealed as the mere offspring
of bodily fear.

But more; the survivors of the conquest might, perhaps, escape, and carry their wasp-fetish into a new land. But if they became poor and weakly, their brains and imagination, degenerating with their bodies, would degrade their wasp-worship till they knew not what it meant. Away from the sacred tree, in a country the wasps of which were not so large or formidable, they would require a remembrancer of the wasp-king; and they would make one—a wasp of wood, or what not. After a while, according to that strange law of fancy, the root of all idolatry, which you may see at work in every child who plays with a doll, the symbol would become identified with the thing symbolised; they would invest the wooden wasp with all the terrible attributes which had belonged to the live wasps of the tree; and after a few centuries, when all remembrance of the tree, the wasp-prophet and chieftain, and his descent from the divine wasp—ay, even of their defeat and flight—had vanished from their songs and legends, they would be found bowing down in fear and trembling to a little ancient wooden wasp, which came from they knew not whence, and meant they knew not what, save that it was a very "old fetish," a "great medicine," or some such other formula for expressing their own ignorance and dread. Just so do the half-savage natives of Thibet, and the Irishwomen of Kerry, by a strange coincidence—unless the ancient Irish were Buddhists, like the Himalayans—tie just the same scraps of rag on the bushes round just the same holy wells, as do the Negros of Central Africa upon their "Devil's Trees;" they know not why, save that their ancestors did it, and it is a charm against ill-luck and danger.

And the sacred tree? That, too, might undergo a metamorphosis in the minds of men. The conquerors would see their aboriginal slaves of the old race still haunting the tree, making stealthy offerings to it by night: and they would ask the reason. But they would not be told. The secret would be guarded; such secrets were guarded, in Greece, in Italy, in medieval France, by the superstitious awe, the cunning, even the hidden self-conceit, of the conquered race. Then the conquerors would wish to imitate their own slaves. They might be in the right. There might be something magical, uncanny, in the hollow tree, which might hurt them; might be jealous of them as intruders. They, too, would invest the place with sacred awe. If they were gloomy, like the Teutonic conquerors of Europe and the Arabian conquerors of the East, they would invest it with unseen terrors. They would say, like them, a devil lives in the tree. If they were of a sunny temper, like the Hellenes, they would invest it with unseen graces. What a noble tree! What a fair fountain hard by its roots! Surely some fair and graceful being must dwell therein, and come out to bathe by night in that clear wave. What meant the fruit, the

flowers, the honey, which the slaves left there by night ?
Pure food for some pure nymph. The wasp-gods would
be forgotten ; probably smoked out as sacrilegious intruders. The lucky seer or poet who struck out the
fancy would soon find imitators ; and it would become,
after a while, a common and popular superstition that
Hamadryads haunted the hollow forest trees, Naiads
the wells, and Oreads the lawns. Somewhat thus, I
presume, did the more cheerful Hellenic myths dis-
place the darker superstitions of the Pelasgi, and those
rude Arcadian tribes who offered, even as late as the
Roman Empire, human sacrifices to gods whose original
names were forgotten.

But even the cultus of nymphs would be defiled after
a while by a darker element. However fair, they
might be capricious and revengeful, like other women.
Why not ? And soon, men going out into the forest
would be missed for a while. They had eaten narcotic
berries, got sun-strokes, wandered till they lost their
wits. At all events, their wits were gone. Who had
done it ? Who but the nymphs ? The men had seen
something they should not have seen ; done something
they would not have done ; and the nymphs had
punished the unconscious rudeness by that frenzy.
Fear, everywhere fear, of Nature—the spotted panther,
as some one calls her, as fair as cruel, as playful as
treacherous. Always fear of Nature, till a Divine light

arise, and show men that they are not the puppets of Nature, but her lords; and that they are to fear God, and fear naught else.

And so ends my true myth of the wasp-tree. No, it need not end there; it may develop into a yet darker and more hideous form of superstition, which Europe has often seen; which is common now among the Negros; * which, we may hope, will soon be exterminated.

This might happen. For it, or something like it, has happened too many times already.

That to the ancient women who still kept up the irrational remnant of the wasp-worship, beneath the sacred tree, other women might resort; not merely from curiosity, or an excited imagination, but from jealousy and revenge. Oppressed, as woman has always been under the reign of brute force; beaten, outraged, deserted, at best married against her will, she has too often gone for comfort and help—and those of the very darkest kind—to the works of darkness; and there never were wanting—there are not wanting, even now, in remote parts of these isles—wicked old women who would, by help of the old superstitions, do for her what she wished. Soon would follow mysterious deaths of

* For an account of Sorcery and Fetishism among the African Negros, see Burton's 'Lake Regions of Central Africa,' vol. ii. pp. 341-360.

rivals, of husbands, of babes; then rumours of dark rites connected with the sacred tree, with poison, with the wasp and his sting, with human sacrifices; lies mingled with truth, more and more confused and frantic, the more they were misinvestigated by men mad with fear: till there would arise one of those witch-manias, which are too common still among the African Negros, which were too common of old among the men of our race.

I say, among the men. To comprehend a witch-mania, you must look at it as—what the witch-literature confesses it unblushingly to be—man's dread of Nature excited to its highest form, as dread of woman.

She is to the barbarous man—she should be more and more to the civilised man—not only the most beautiful and precious, but the most wonderful and mysterious of all natural objects, if it be only as the author of his physical being. She is to the savage a miracle to be alternately adored and dreaded. He dreads her more delicate nervous organisation, which often takes shapes to him demoniacal and miraculous; her quicker instincts, her readier wit, which seem to him to have in them somewhat prophetic and super-human, which entangle him as in an invisible net, and rule him against his will. He dreads her very tongue, more crushing than his heaviest club, more keen than his poisoned arrows. He dreads those habits of secresy and falsehood, the weapons of the weak, to which savage and degraded woman always has recourse. He dreads the very medicinal skill which she has learnt to exercise, as nurse, comforter, and slave. He dreads those secret ceremonies, those mysterious initiations which no man may witness, which he has permitted to her in all ages, in so many—if not all—barbarous and semi-barbarous races, whether Negro, American, Syrian, Greek, or Roman, as a homage to the mysterious importance of her who brings him into the world. If she turn against him—she, with all her unknown powers, she who is the sharer of his deepest secrets, who prepares his very food day by day —what harm can she not, may she not do? And that she has good reason to turn against him, he knows too well. What deliverance is there from this mysterious house-fiend, save brute force? Terror, torture, murder, must be the order of the day. Woman must be crushed, at all price, by the blind fear of the man.

I shall say no more. I shall draw a veil, for very pity and shame, over the most important and most significant facts of this, the most hideous of all human follies. I have, I think, given you hints enough to show that it, like all other superstitions, is the child— the last born and the ugliest child—of blind dread of the unknown.

SCIENCE.

A LECTURE DELIVERED AT THE ROYAL INSTITUTION.

———◦◦◦———

I SAID, that Superstition was the child of Fear, and Fear the child of Ignorance; and you might expect me to say antithetically, that Science was the child of Courage, and Courage the child of Knowledge.

But these genealogies—like most metaphors—do not fit exactly, as you may see for yourselves.

If fear be the child of ignorance, ignorance is also the child of fear; the two react on, and produce each other. The more men dread Nature, the less they wish to know about her. Why pry into her awful secrets? It is dangerous; perhaps impious. She says to them, as in the Egyptian temple of old—"I am Isis, and my veil no mortal yet hath lifted." And why should they try or wish to lift it? If she will leave them in peace, they will leave her in peace. It is enough that she does not destroy them. So as ignorance bred fear, fear breeds fresh and willing ignorance.

And courage? We may say, and truly, that courage is the child of knowledge. But we may say as truly, that knowledge is the child of courage. Those Egyptian priests in the temple of Isis would have told you that knowledge was the child of mystery, of special illumination, of reverence, and what not; hiding under grand words their purpose of keeping the masses ignorant, that they might be their slaves. Reverence? I will yield to none in reverence for reverence. I will all but agree with the wise man who said that reverence is the root of all virtues. But which child reverences his father most? He who comes joyfully and trustfully to meet him, that he may learn his father's mind, and do his will: or he who at his father's coming runs away and hides, lest he should be beaten. for he knows not what? There is a scientific reverence, a reverence of courage, which is surely one of the highest forms of reverence. That, namely, which so reveres every fact, that it dare not overlook or falsify it, seem it never so minute; which feels that because it is a fact, it cannot be minute, cannot be unimportant; that it must be a fact of God; a message from God; a voice of God, as Bacon has it, revealed in things; and which therefore, just because it stands in solemn awe of such paltry facts as the Scolopax feather in a snipe's pinion, or the jagged leaves which appear capriciously in certain honeysuckles, believes

that there is likely to be some deep and wide secret
underlying them, which is worth years of thought to
solve. That is reverence; a reverence which is growing, thank God, more and more common; which will
produce, as it grows more common still, fruit which
generations yet unborn shall bless.

But as for that other reverence, which shuts its eyes
and ears in pious awe—what is it but cowardice decked
out in state robes, putting on the sacred Urim and Thum-
mim, not that men may ask counsel of the Deity, but
that they may not? What is it but cowardice, very
pitiable when unmasked; and what is its child but ignorance as pitiable, which would be ludicrous were it not
so injurious? If a man comes up to Nature as to a
parrot or a monkey, with this prevailing thought in
his head—Will it bite me?—will he not be pretty certain to make up his mind that it may bite him, and
had therefore best be left alone? It is only the man
of courage—few and far between—who will stand the
chance of a first bite, in the hope of teaching the parrot
to talk, or the monkey to fire off a gun. And it is only
the man of courage—few and far between—who will
stand the chance of a first bite from Nature, which may
kill him for aught he knows—for her teeth, though
clumsy, are very strong—in order that he may tame
her and break her in to his use by the very same
method by which that admirable inductive philosopher,

Mr. Rarey, used to break in his horses; first, by not being afraid of them; and next, by trying to find out what they were thinking of. But after all, as with animals, so with Nature; cowardice is dangerous. The surest method of getting bitten by an animal is to be afraid of it; and the surest method of being injured by Nature is to be afraid of it. Only as far as we understand Nature are we safe from it; and those who in any age counsel mankind not to pry into the secrets of the universe, counsel them not to provide for their own life and well-being, or for their children after them.

But how few there have been in any age who have not been afraid of Nature. How few have set themselves, like Rarey, to tame her by finding out what she is thinking of. The mass are glad to have the results of science, as they are to buy Mr. Rarey's horses after they are tamed: but for want of courage or of wit, they had rather leave the taming process to some one else. And therefore we may say that what knowledge of Nature we have—and we have very little— we owe to the courage of those men—and they have been very few—who have been inspired to face Nature boldly; and say—or, what is better, act as if they were saying—"I find something in me which I do not find in you; which gives me the hope that I can grow to understand you, though you may not understand me; that I may become your master, and not as now, you mine. And if not, I will know: or die in the search."

It is to those men, the few and far between, in a very few ages and very few countries, who have thus risen in rebellion against Nature, and looked it in the face with an unquailing glance, that we owe what we call Physical Science.

There have been four races—or rather a very few men of each four races—who have faced Nature after this gallant wise.

First, the old Jews. I speak of them, be it remembered, exclusively from an historical, and not a religious point of view.

These people, at a very remote epoch, emerged from a country highly civilised, but sunk in the superstitions of nature-worship. They invaded and mingled with tribes whose superstitions were even more debased, silly, and foul than those of the Egyptians from whom they escaped. Their own masses were for centuries given up to nature-worship. Now among those Jews arose men—a very few—sages—prophets—call them what you will, the men were inspired heroes and philosophers—who assumed towards nature an attitude utterly different from the rest of their countrymen and the rest of the then world; who denounced superstition and the dread of nature as the parent of all manner of vice and misery; who for themselves said boldly that

they discerned in the universe an order, a unity, a per-
manence of law, which gave them courage instead of
fear. They found delight and not dread in the thought
that the universe obeyed a law which could not be
broken; that all things continued to that day according to a certain ordinance. They took a view of Nature
totally new in that age; healthy, human, cheerful,
loving, trustful, and yet reverent—identical with that
which happily is beginning to prevail in our own day.
They defied those very volcanic and meteoric phenomena of their land, to which their countrymen were
slaying their own children in the clefts of the rocks,
and, like Theophrastus' superstitious man, pouring their
drink-offerings on the smooth stones of the valley;
and declared that, for their part, they would not fear,
though the earth was moved, and though the hills were
carried into the midst of the sea; though the waters
raged and swelled, and the mountains shook at the
tempest.

The fact is indisputable. And you must pardon me
if I express my belief that these men, if they had felt
it their business to found a school of inductive physical
science, would, owing to that temper of mind, have
achieved a very signal success. I ground that opinion
on the remarkable, but equally indisputable fact, that
no nation has ever succeeded in perpetuating a school
of inductive physical science, save those whose minds

have been saturated with this same view of Nature, which they have—as an historic fact—slowly but thoroughly learnt from the writings of these Jewish sages.

Such is the fact. The founders of inductive physical science were not the Jews: but first the Chaldæans, next the Greeks, next their pupils the Romans—or rather a few sages among each race. But what success had they? The Chaldæan astronomers made a few discoveries concerning the motions of the heavenly bodies, which, rudimentary as they were, still prove them to have been men of rare intellect. For a great and a patient genius must he have been, who first distinguished the planets from the fixed stars, or worked out the earliest astronomical caclulation. But they seem to have been crushed, as it were, by their own discoveries. They stopped short. They gave way again to the primeval fear of Nature. They sank into planet-worship. They invented, it would seem, that fantastic pseudo-science of astrology, which lay for ages after as an incubus on the human intellect and conscience. They became the magicians and quacks of the old world; and mankind owed them thenceforth nothing but evil. Among the Greeks and Romans, again, those sages who dared face Nature like reasonable men, were accused by the superstitious mob as irreverent, impious atheists. The wisest of them all, Socrates, was actually put to death on that charge; and finally, they

failed. School after school, in Greece and Rome, struggled to discover, and to get a hearing for, some theory
of the universe which was founded on something like
experience, reason, common sense. They were not
allowed to prosecute their attempt. The mud-ocean
of ignorance and fear in which they struggled so
manfully was too strong for them; the mud-waves
closed over their heads finally, as the age of the Anto-
nines expired; and the last effort of Græco-Roman
thought to explain the universe was Neoplatonism—
the muddiest of the muddy—an attempt to apologise
for, and organise into a system, all the nature-dreading
superstitions of the Roman world. Porphyry, Plotinus,
Proclus, poor Hypatia herself, and all her school—they
may have had themselves no bodily fear of Nature; for
they were noble souls. Yet they spent their time in
justifying those who had; in apologising for the superstitions of the very mob which they despised: just as—
it sometimes seems to me—some folk in these days are
like to end in doing; begging that the masses might be
allowed to believe in anything, however false, lest they
should believe in nothing at all: as if believing in lies
could do anything but harm to any human being. And
so died the science of the old world, in a true second
childhood, just where it began.

The Jewish sages, I hold, taught that science was
probable; the Greeks and Romans proved that it was

possible. It remained for our race, under the teaching of both, to bring science into act and fact.

Many causes contributed to give them this power. They were a personally courageous race. This earth has yet seen no braver men than the forefathers of Christian Europe, whether Scandinavian or Teuton, Angle or Frank. They were a practical hard-headed race, with a strong appreciation of facts, and a strong determination to act on them. Their laws, their society, their commerce, their colonisation, their migrations by land and sea, proved that they were such. They were favoured, moreover, by circumstances, or—as I should rather put it—by that divine Providence which determined their times, and the bounds of their habitation. They came in as the heritors of the decaying civilisation of Greece and Rome; they colonised territories which gave to man special fair play, but no more, in the struggle for existence, the battle with the powers of Nature; tolerably fertile, tolerably temperate; with boundless means of water communication; freer than most parts of the world from those terrible natural phenomena, like the earthquake and the hurricane, before which man lies helpless and astounded, a child beneath the foot of a giant. Nature was to them not so inhospitable as to starve their brains and limbs, as it has done for the Esquimaux or Fuegian; and not so bountiful as to crush them by its very luxuriance,

as it has crushed the savages of the tropics. They
saw enough of its strength to respect it; not enough
to cower before it: and they and it have fought it out;
and it seems to me, standing either on London Bridge
or on a Holland fen-dyke, that they are winning at last.

But they had a sore battle: a battle against their
own fear of the unseen. They brought with them, out
of the heart of Asia, dark and sad nature-superstitions,
some of which linger among our peasantry till this day,
of elves, trolls, nixes, and what not. Their Thor and
Odin were at first, probably, only the thunder and the
wind: but they had to be appeased in the dark marches
of the forest, where hung rotting on the sacred oaks,
amid carcases of goat and horse, the carcases of human
victims. No one acquainted with the early legends
and ballads of our race, but must perceive throughout
them all the prevailing tone of fear and sadness. And
to their own superstitions they added those of the
Rome which they conquered. They dreaded the Roman
she-poisoners and witches, who, like Horace's Canidia,
still performed horrid rites in grave-yards and dark
places of the earth. They dreaded as magical the
delicate images engraved on old Greek gems. They
dreaded the very Roman cities they had destroyed.
They were the work of enchanters. Like the ruins of
St. Albans here in England, they were all full of devils,
guarding the treasures which the Romans had hidden.

The Cæsars became to them magical man-gods. The poet Virgil became the prince of necromancers. If the secrets of Nature were to be known, they were to be known by unlawful means, by prying into the mysteries of the old heathen magicians, or of the Mohammedan doctors of Cordova and Seville; and those who dared to do so were respected and feared, and often came to evil ends. It needed moral courage, then, to face and interpret fact. Such brave men as Pope Gerbert, Roger Bacon, Galileo, even Kepler, did not lead happy lives; some of them found themselves in prison. All the medieval sages — even Albertus Magnus — were stigmatised as magicians. One wonders that more of them did not imitate poor Paracelsus, who, unable to get a hearing for his coarse common sense, took—vain and sensual—to drinking the laudanum which he him-self had discovered, and vaunted as a priceless boon to men; and died as the fool dieth, in spite of all his wisdom. For the "Romani nominis umbra," the shadow of the mighty race whom they had conquered, lay heavy on our forefathers for centuries. And their dread of the great heathens was really a dread of Nature, and of the powers thereof. For when the authority of great names has reigned unquestioned for many centuries, those names become, to the human mind, integral and necessary parts of Nature itself. They are, as it were, absorbed into it; they become its laws, its canons, its demiurges, and guardian spirits; their words become regarded as actual facts; in one word, they become a superstition, and are feared as parts of the vast unknown; and to deny what they have said is, in the minds of the many, not merely to fly in the face of reverent wisdom, but to fly in the face of facts. During a great part of the middle ages, for instance, it was impossible for an educated man to think of Nature itself, without thinking first of what Aristotle had said of her. Aristotle's dicta were Nature; and when Benedetti, at Venice, opposed in 1585 Aristotle's opinions on violent and natural motion, there were hundreds, perhaps, in the universities of Europe—as there certainly were in the days of the immortal 'Epistolæ Obscurorum Virorum '—who were ready, in spite of all Benedetti's professed reverence for Aristotle, to accuse him of outraging not only the father of philosophy, but Nature itself and its palpable and notorious facts. For the restoration of letters in the fifteenth century had not at first mended matters, so strong was the dread of Nature in the minds of the masses. The minds of men had sported forth, not toward any sound investigation of facts, but toward an eclectic resuscitation of Neoplatonism; which endured, not without a certain beauty and use—as let Spenser's 'Faery Queen' bear witness—till the latter half of the seventeenth century.

After that time a rapid change began. It is marked by—it has been notably assisted by—the foundation of our own Royal Society. Its causes I will not enter into ; they are so inextricably mixed, I hold, with theological questions, that they cannot be discussed here. I will only point out to you these facts : that, from the latter part of the seventeenth century, the noblest heads and the noblest hearts of Europe concentrated themselves more and more on the brave and patient investigation of physical facts, as the source of priceless future blessings to mankind ; that the eighteenth century, which it has been the fashion of late to depreciate, did more for the welfare of mankind, in every conceivable direction, than the whole fifteen centuries before it ; that it did this good work by boldly observing and analysing facts ; that this boldness towards facts increased in proportion as Europe became indoctrinated with the Jewish literature ; and that, notably, such men as Kepler, Newton, Berkeley, Spinoza, Leibnitz, Descartes, in whatsoever else they differed, agreed in this, that their attitude towards Nature was derived from the teaching of the Jewish sages. I believe that we are not yet fully aware how much we owe to the Jewish mind, in the gradual emancipation of the human intellect. The connection may not, of course, be one of cause and effect ; it may be a mere coincidence. I believe it to be a cause ; one of course of very many causes: but still an integral cause. At least the coincidence is too remarkable a fact not to be worthy of investigation.

I said, just now—The emancipation of the human intellect. I did not say—Of science, or of the scientific intellect; and for this reason:

That the emancipation of science is the emancipation of the common mind of all men. All men can partake of the gains of free scientific thought, not merely by enjoying its physical results, but by becoming more scientific men themselves.

Therefore it was, that though I began my first lecture by defining superstition, I did not begin my second by defining its antagonist, science. For the word science defines itself. It means simply knowledge; that is, of course right knowledge, or such an approximation as can be obtained; knowledge of any natural object, its classification, its causes, its effects; or in plain English, what it is, how it came where it is, and what can be done with it.

And scientific method, likewise, needs no definition; for it is simply the exercise of common sense. It is not a peculiar, unique, professional, or mysterious process of the understanding: but the same which all men employ, from the cradle to the grave, in forming correct conclusions.

Every one who knows the philosophic writings of

Mr. John Stuart Mill, will be familiar with this opinion. But to those who have no leisure to study him, I should recommend the reading of Professor Huxley's third lecture on the origin of species.

In that he shows, with great logical skill, as well as with some humour, how the man who, on rising in the morning, finds the parlour window open, the spoons and teapot gone, the mark of a dirty hand on the window-sill, and that of a hob-nailed boot outside, and comes to the conclusion that some one has broken open the window, and stolen the plate, arrives at that hypo- thesis—for it is nothing more—by a long and complex train of inductions and deductions, of just the same kind as those which, according to the Baconian philo- sophy, are to be used for investigating the deepest secrets of Nature.

This is true, even of those sciences which involve long mathematical calculations. In fact, the stating of the problem to be solved is the most important element in the calculation; and that is so thoroughly a labour of common sense that an utterly uneducated man may, and often does, state an abstruse problem clearly and correctly; seeing what ought to be proved, and perhaps how to prove it, though he may be unable to work the problem out, for want of mathematical knowledge

But that mathematical knowledge is not—as all Cambridge men are surely aware—the result of any

T

special gift. It is merely the development of those conceptions of form and number which every human being possesses; and any person of average intellect can make himself a fair mathematician if he will only pay continuous attention; in plain English, think enough about the subject.

There are sciences, again, which do not involve mathematical calculation; for instance, botany, zoology, geology, which are just now passing from their old stage of classificatory sciences into the rank of organic ones. These are, without doubt, altogether within the scope of the merest common sense. Any man or woman of average intellect, if they will but observe and think for themselves, freely, boldly, patiently, accurately, may judge for themselves of the conclusions of these sciences, may add to these conclusions fresh and important discoveries; and if I am asked for a proof of what I assert, I point to 'Rain and Rivers,' written by no professed scientific man, but by a colonel in the Guards, known to fame only as one of the most perfect horsemen in the world.

Let me illustrate my meaning by an example. A man—I do not say a geologist, but simply a man, squire or ploughman—sees a small valley, say one of the side-glens which open into the larger valleys in the Windsor forest district. He wishes to ascertain its age.

He has, at first sight, a very simple measure—that of denudation. He sees that the glen is now being eaten out by a little stream, the product of innumerable springs which arise along its sides, and which are fed entirely by the rain on the moors above. He finds, on observation, that this stream brings down some ten cubic yards of sand and gravel, on an average, every year. The actual quantity of earth which has been removed to make the glen may be several million cubic yards. Here is an easy sum in arithmetic. At the rate of ten cubic yards a year, the stream has taken several hundred thousand years to make the glen.

You will observe that this result is obtained by mere common sense. He has a right to assume that the stream originally began the glen, because he finds it in the act of enlarging it; just as much right as he has to assume, if he find a hole in his pocket, and his last coin in the act of falling through it, that the rest of his money has fallen through the same hole. It is a sufficient cause, and the simplest. A number of observations as to the present rate of denudation, and a sum which any railroad contractor can do in his head, to determine the solid contents of the valley, are all that are needed. The method is that of science : but it is also that of simple common sense. You will remember, therefore, that this is no mere theory or hypothesis, but a pretty fair and simple conclusion from palpable facts; that the probability lies with the belief that the glen is some hundreds of thousands of years old ; that it is not the observer's business to prove it further, but other persons' to disprove it, if they can.

But does the matter end here? No. And, for certain reasons, it is good that it should not end here.

The observer, if he be a cautious man, begins to see if he can disprove his own conclusions ; moreover, being human, he is probably somewhat awed, if not appalled, by his own conclusion. Hundreds of thousands of years spent in making that little glen ! Common sense would say that the longer it took to make, the less wonder there was in its being made at last : but the instinctive human feeling is the opposite. There is in men, and there remains in them, even after they are civilised, and all other forms of the dread of Nature have died out in them, a dread of size, of vast space, of vast time; that latter, mind, being always imagined as space, as we confess when we speak instinctively of a space of time. They will not understand that size is merely a relative, not an absolute term; that if we were a thousand times larger than we are, the universe would be a thousand times smaller than it is; that if we could think a thousand times faster than we do, time would be a thousand times longer than it is; that there is One in whom we live, and move, and have our being, to whom one day is as a thousand years, and a thousand years as one day. I believe this dread of size to be merely, like all other superstitions, a result of bodily fear ; a development of the instinct which makes a little dog run away from a big dog. Be that as it may, every observer has it; and so the man's conclusion seems to him strange, doubtful : he will reconsider it.

Moreover, if he be an experienced man, he is well aware that first guesses, first hypotheses, are not always the right ones ; and if he be a modest man, he will consider the fact that many thousands of thoughtful men in all ages, and many thousands still, would say, that the glen can only be a few thousand, or possibly a few hundred, years old. And he will feel bound to consider their opinion ; as far as it is, like his own, drawn from facts, but no further.

So he casts about for all other methods by which the glen may have been produced, to see if any one of them will account for it in a shorter time.

1. Was it made by an earthquake ? No; for the strata on both sides are identical, at the same level, and in the same plane.

2. Or by a mighty current ? If so, the flood must have run in at the upper end, before it ran out at the lower. But nothing has run in at the upper end. All round above are the undisturbed gravel beds of the horizontal moor, without channel or depression.

3. Or by water draining off a vast flat as it was upheaved out of the sea ? That is a likely guess. The valley at its upper end spreads out like the fingers of a hand, as the gullies in tide-muds do.

But that hypothesis will not stand. There is no vast unbroken flat behind the glen. Right and left of it are other similar glens, parted from it by long narrow ridges: these also must be explained on the same hypothesis; but they cannot. For there could not have been surface-drainage to make them all, or a tenth of them. There are no other possible hypotheses; and so he must fall back on the original theory—the rain, the springs, the brook; they have done it all, even as they are doing it this day.

But is not that still a hasty assumption ? May not their denuding power have been far greater in old times than now?

Why should it ? Because there was more rain then than now? That he must put out of court; there is no evidence of it whatsoever.

Because the land was more friable originally? Well, there is a great deal to be said for that. The experience of every countryman tells him that bare or fallow land is more easily washed away than land under vegetation. And no doubt, when these gravels and sands rose from the sea, they were barren for hundreds of years. He has some measure of the time required, because he can tell roughly how long it takes for sands and shingles left by the sea to become covered with vegetation. But he must allow that the friability of the land must have been originally much greater than now, for hundreds of years.

But again, does that fact really cut off any great space of time from his hundreds of thousands of years? For when the land first rose from the sea, that glen was not there. Some slight bay or bend in the shore determined its site. That stream was not there. It was split up into a million little springs, oozing side by side from the shore, and having each a very minute denuding power, which kept continually increasing by combination as the glen ate its way inwards, and the rainfall drained by all these little springs was collected into the one central stream. So that when the ground being bare was most liable to be denuded, the water was least able to do it; and as the denuding power of the water increased, the land, being covered with vegetation, became more and more able to resist it. All this he has seen, going on at the present day, in the similar gullies worn in the soft strata of the South Hampshire coast; especially round Bournemouth.

So the two disturbing elements in the calculation may be fairly set off against each other, as making a difference of only a few thousands or tens of thousands of years either way; and the age of the glen may fairly be, if not a million years, yet such a length of years as mankind still speak of with bated breath, as if forsooth it would do them some harm.

I trust that every scientific man in this room will agree with me, that the imaginary squire or plough-man would have been conducting his investigation strictly according to the laws of the Baconian philo-sophy. You will remark, meanwhile, that he has not used a single scientific term, or referred to a single scientific investigation ; and has observed nothing and thought nothing which might not have been observed and thought by any one who chose to use his common sense, and not to be afraid.

But because he has come round, after all this further investigation, to something very like his first conclusion, was all that further investigation useless ? No—a thou-sand times, no. It is this very verification of hypotheses which makes the sound ones safe, and destroys the unsound. It is this struggle with all sorts of super-stitions which makes science strong and sure, and her march irresistible, winning ground slowly, but never receding from it. It is this buffeting of adversity which compels her not to rest dangerously upon the shallow sand of first guesses, and single observations ; but to strike her roots down, deep, wide, and interlaced, into the solid ground of actual facts.

It is very necessary to insist on this point. For

there have been men in all past ages—I do not say whether there are any such now, but I am inclined to think that there will be hereafter—men who have tried to represent scientific method as something difficult, mysterious, peculiar, unique, not to be attained by the unscientific mass; and this not for tho purpose of exalting science, but rather of discrediting her. For as long as the masses, educated or uneducated, are ignorant of what scientific method is, they will look on scientific men, as the middle age looked on necromancers, as a privileged, but awful and uncanny caste, possessed of mighty secrets; who may do them great good, but may also do them great harm.

Which belief on the part of the masses will enable these persons to instal themselves as the critics of science, though not scientific men themselves: and—as Shakespeare has it—to talk of Robin Hood, though they never shot in his bow. Thus they become mediators to the masses between the scientific and the unscientific worlds. They tell them—You are not to trust the conclusions of men of science at first hand. You are not fit judges of their facts or of their methods. It is we who will, by a cautious eclecticism, choose out for you such of their conclusions as are safe for you; and them we will advise you to believe. To the scientific man, on the other hand, as often as anything is discovered unpleasing to them, they will say, imperiously and e cathedrâ—Your new theory contradicts the esta‑blished facts of science. For they will know well that whatever the men of science think of their assertion, the masses will believe it; totally unaware that the speakers are by their very terms showing their igno‑rance of science; and that what they call established facts scientific men call merely provisional conclusions, which they would throw away to-morrow without a pang were the known facts explained better by a fresh theory, or did fresh facts require one.

This has happened too often. It is in the interest of superstition that it should happen again; and the best way to prevent it surely is to tell the masses—Scientific method is no peculiar mystery, requiring a peculiar initiation. It is simply common sense, com‑bined with uncommon courage, which includes uncom‑mon honesty and uncommon patience; and if you will be brave, honest, patient, and rational, you will need no mystagogues to tell you what in science to believe and what not to believe; for you will be just as good judges of scientific facts and theories as those who assume the right of guiding your convictions. You are men and women: and more than that you need not be.

And let me say that the man of our days whose writings exemplify most thoroughly what I am going to say is the justly revered Mr. Thomas Carlyle.

As far as I know he has never written on any scien‑

tific subject. For aught I am aware of, he may know nothing of mathematics or chemistry, of comparative anatomy or geology. For aught I am aware of, he may know a great deal about them all, and, like a wise man, hold his tongue, and give the world merely the results in the form of general thought. But this I know; that his writings are instinct with the very spirit of science; that he has taught men, more than any living man, the meaning and end of science; that he has taught men moral and intellectual courage; to face facts boldly, while they confess the divineness of facts; not to be afraid of Nature, and not to worship nature; to believe that man can know truth; and that only in as far as he knows truth can he live worthily on this earth. And thus he has vindicated, as no other man in our days has done, at once the dignity of Nature and the dignity of spirit. That he would have made a distinguished scientific man, we may be as certain from his writings as we may be certain, when we seen a fine old horse of a certain stamp, that he would have made a first-class hunter, though he has been unfortunately all his life in harness. Therefore, did I try to train a young man of science to be true, devout, and earnest, accurate and daring, I should say—Read what you will: but at least read Carlyle. It is a small matter to me—and I doubt not to him—whether you will agree with his special conclusions: but his premises and

his method are irrefragable ; for they stand on the
"voluntatem Dei in rebus revelatam"—on fact and
common sense.

And Mr. Carlyle's writings, if I am correct in my
estimate of them, will afford a very sufficient answer
to those who think that the scientific habit of mind
tends to irreverence.

Doubtless this accusation will always be brought
against science by those who confound reverence with
fear.   For from blind fear of the unknown, science does
certainly deliver man.   She does by man as he does
by an unbroken colt.   The colt sees by the road side
some quite new object—a cast-away boot, an old kettle,
or what not.   What a fearful monster !   What unknown
terrific powers may it not possess !   And the colt
shies across the road, runs up the bank, rears on end ;
putting itself thereby, as many a man does, in real
danger.   What cure is there ?   But one ; experience.
So science takes us, as we should take the colt, gently
by the halter ; and makes us simply smell at the new
monster ; till after a few trembling sniffs, we discover,
like the colt, that it is not a monster, but a kettle.
Yet I think, if we sum up the loss and gain, we shall
find the colt's character has gained, rather than lost,
by being thus disabused.   He learns to substitute a
very rational reverence for the man who is breaking
him in, for a totally irrational reverence for the kettle ;

and becomes thereby a much wiser and more useful member of society, as does the man when disabused of his superstitions.

From which follows one result. That if science proposes—as she does—to make men brave, wise, and independent, she must needs excite unpleasant feelings in all who desire to keep men cowardly, ignorant, and slavish. And that too many such persons have existed in all ages is but too notorious. There have been from all time, goëtai, quacks, powwow men, rain-makers, and necromancers of various sorts, who having for their own purposes set forth partial, ill-grounded, fantastic, and frightful interpretations of nature, have no love for those who search after a true, exact, brave, and hopeful one. And therefore it is to be feared, or hoped, science and superstition will to the world's end remain irreconcilable and internecine foes.

Conceive the feelings of an old Lapland witch, who has had for the last fifty years all the winds in a seal-skin bag, and has been selling fair breezes to northern skippers at so much a puff, asserting her powers so often, poor old soul, that she has got to half believe them herself,—conceive, I say, her feelings at seeing her customers watch the Admiralty storm-signals, and con the weather reports in the 'Times.' Conceive the feelings of Sir Samuel Baker's African friend, Katchiba, the rain-making chief, who possessed a whole housefull

of thunder and lightning—though he did not, he confessed, keep it in a bottle as they do in England—if
Sir Samuel had had the means, and the will, of giving
to Katchiba's Negros a course of lectures on electricity, with appropriate experiments, and a real bottle
full of real lightning among the foremost.

It is clear that only two methods of self-defence
would have been open to the rain-maker : namely, either
to kill Sir Samuel, or to buy his real secret of bottling
the lightning, that he might use it for his own ends.
The former method—that of killing the man of science—
was found more easy in ancient times ; the latter in
these modern ones. And there have been always those
who, too good-natured to kill the scientific man, have
patronised knowledge, not for its own sake, but for the
use which may be made of it ; who would like to keep
a tame man of science, as they would a tame poet, or a
tame parrot ; who say—Let us have science by all
means, but not too much of it. It is a dangerous
thing ; to be doled out to the world, like medicine,
in small and cautious doses. You, the scientific man,
will of course freely discover what you choose. Only
do not talk too loudly about it : leave that to us. We
understand the world, and are meant to guide and
govern it. So discover freely : and meanwhile hand
over your discoveries to us, that we may instruct and
edify the populace with so much of them as we think

safe, while we keep our position thereby, and in many
cases make much money by your science. Do that,
and we will patronise you, applaud you, ask you to our
houses; and you shall be clothed in purple and fine
linen, and fare sumptuously with us every day. I
know not whether these latter are not the worst enemies which science has. They are often such excellent,
respectable, orderly, well-meaning persons. They desire so sincerely that everyone should be wise: only not
too wise. They are so utterly unaware of the mischief
they are doing. They would recoil with horror if they
were told they were so many Iscariots, betraying Truth
with a kiss.

But science, as yet, has withstood both terrors and
blandishments. In old times, she endured being imprisoned and slain. She came to life again. Perhaps
it was the will of Him in whom all things live, that
she should live. Perhaps it was His spirit which gave
her life.

She can endure, too, being starved. Her votaries
have not as yet cared much for purple and fine linen,
and sumptuous fare. There are a very few among
them who, joining brilliant talents to solid learning,
have risen to deserved popularity, to titles, and to
wealth. But even their labours, it seems to me, are
never rewarded in any proportion to the time and the
intellect spent on them, nor to the benefits which they

bring to mankind; while the great majority, unpaid and unknown, toil on, and have to find in science her own reward. Better, perhaps, that it should be so. Better for science that she should be free, in holy poverty, to go where she will and say what she knows, than that she should be hired out at so much a year to say things pleasing to the many, and to those who guide the many. And so, I verily believe, the majority of scientific men think. There are those among them who have obeyed very faithfully St. Paul's precept, "No man that warreth entangleth himself with the affairs of this life." For they have discovered that they are engaged in a war—a veritable war—against the rulers of darkness, against ignorance and its twin children, fear and cruelty. Of that war they see neither the end nor even the plan. But they are ready to go on; ready, with Socrates, "to follow reason whithersoever it leads;" and content, meanwhile, like good soldiers in a campaign, if they can keep tolerably in line, and use their weapons, and see a few yards ahead of them through the smoke and the woods. They will come out somewhere at last; they know not where nor when: but they will come out at last, into the daylight and the open field; and be told then—perhaps to their own astonishment—as many a gallant soldier has been told, that by simply walking straight on, and doing the duty which lay nearest them, they have helped to win a great battle, and slay great giants, earning the thanks of their country and of mankind.

And, meanwhile, if they get their shilling a day of fighting-pay, they are content. I had almost said, they ought to be content. For science is, I verily believe, like virtue, its own exceeding great reward. I can conceive few human states more enviable than that of the man to whom, panting in the foul laboratory, or watching for his life under the tropic forest, Isis shall for a moment lift her sacred veil, and show him, once and for ever, the thing he dreamed not of; some law, or even mere hint of a law, explaining one fact; but explaining with it a thousand more, connecting them all with each other and with the mighty whole, till order and meaning shoots through some old Chaos of scattered observations.

Is not that a joy, a prize, which wealth cannot give, nor poverty take away? What it may lead to, he knows not. Of what use it may become, he knows not. But this he knows, that somewhere it must lead; of some use it will be. For it is a truth; and having found a truth, he has exorcised one more of the ghosts which haunt humanity. He has left one object less for man to fear; one object more for man to use. Yes, the scientific man may have this comfort, that whatever he has done, he has done good; that he is

U

following a mistress who has never yet conferred aught but benefits on the human race.

What physical science may do hereafter I know not; but as yet she has done this:

She has enormously increased the wealth of the human race; and has therefore given employment, food, existence, to millions who, without science, would either have starved or have never been born. She has shown that the dictum of the early political economists, that population has a tendency to increase faster than the means of subsistence, is no law of humanity, but merely a tendency of the barbaric and ignorant man, which can be counteracted by increasing manifold by scientific means his powers of producing food. She has taught men, during the last few years, to foresee and elude the most destructive storms; and there is no reason for doubting, and many reasons for hoping, that she will gradually teach men to elude other terrific forces of nature, too powerful and too seemingly capricious for them to conquer. She has discovered innumerable remedies and alleviations for pains and disease. She has thrown such light on the causes of epidemics, that we are able to say now that the presence of cholera—and probably of all zymotic diseases—in any place, is usually a sin and a shame, for which the owners and authorities of that place ought to be punishable by law, as destroyers of their fellow-men;

---

while for the weak, for those who, in the barbarous and semi-barbarous state—and out of that last we are only just emerging—how much has she done ; an earnest of much more which she will do ? She has delivered the insane—I may say by the scientific insight of one man, more worthy of titles and pensions than nine-tenths of those who earn them—I mean the great and good Pinel —from hopeless misery and torture into comparative peace and comfort, and at least the possibility of cure. For children, she has done much, or rather might do, would parents read and perpend such books as Andrew Combe's and those of other writers on physical education. We should not then see the children, even of the rich, done to death piecemeal by improper food, improper clothes, neglect of ventilation and the commonest measures for preserving health. We should not see their intellects stunted by Procrustean attempts to teach them all the same accomplishments, to the neglect, most often, of any sound practical training of their faculties. We should not see slight indigestion, or temporary rushes of blood to the head, condemned and punished as sins against Him who took up little children in His arms and blessed them.

But we may have hope. When we compare education now with what it was even forty years ago, much more with the stupid brutality of the monastic system, we may hail for children, as well as for grown people, the advent of the reign of common sense.

And for woman—What might I not say on that point? But most of it would be fitly discussed only among physicians and biologists: here I will say only this—Science has exterminated, at least among civilised nations, witch-manias. Women—at least white women —are no longer tortured or burnt alive from man's blind fear of the unknown. If science had done no more than that, she would deserve the perpetual thanks and the perpetual trust, not only of the women whom she has preserved from agony, but the men whom she has preserved from crime.

These benefits have already accrued to civilised men, because they have lately allowed a very few of their number peaceably to imitate Mr. Rarey, and find out what nature—or rather, to speak at once reverently and accurately, He who made nature—is thinking of; and obey the "voluntatem Dei in rebus revelatam." This science has done, while yet in her infancy. What she will do in her maturity, who dare predict? At least, in the face of such facts as these, those who bid us fear, or restrain, or mutilate science, bid us commit an act of folly, as well as of ingratitude, which can only harm ourselves. For science has as yet done nothing but good. Will any one tell me what harm it has ever done? When any one will show me a single result of science, of the knowledge of and use of physical facts, which has not tended directly to the benefit of mankind, moral and spiritual, as well as physical and economic— then I shall be tempted to believe that Solomon was wrong when he said that the one thing to be sought after on earth, more precious than all treasure, she who has length of days in her right hand, and in her left hand riches and honour, whose ways are ways of pleasantness and all her paths are peace, who is a tree of life to all who lay hold on her, and makes happy every one who retains her, is—as you will see if you will yourselves consult the passage—that very Wisdom —by which God has founded the earth; and that very Understanding—by which He has established the heavens.

GROTS AND GROVES.

I wish this lecture to be suggestive, rather than didactic; to set you thinking and inquiring for yourselves, rather than learning at second-hand from me. Some among my audience, I doubt not, will neither need to be taught by me, nor to be stirred up to inquiry for themselves. They are already, probably, antiquarians; already better acquainted with the subject than I am. They come hither, therefore, as critics; I trust not as unkindly critics. They will, I hope, remember that I am trying to excite a general interest in that very architecture in which they delight, and so to make the public do justice to their labours. They will therefore, I trust,

> " Be to my faults a little blind,
> Be to my virtues very kind ; "

and if my architectural theories do not seem to them correct in all details—well-founded I believe them myself to be—remember that it is a slight matter to me, or to the audience, whether any special and pet fancy of mine should be exactly true or not: but it is not a light matter that my hearers should be awakened —and too many just now need an actual awakening—to a right, pure, and wholesome judgment on questions of art, especially when the soundness of that judgment depends, as in this case, on sound judgments about human history, as well as about natural objects.

Now, it befel me that, fresh from the Tropic forests, and with their forms hanging always, as it were, in the background of my eye, I was impressed more and more vividly the longer I looked, with the likeness of those forest forms to the forms of our own Cathedral of Chester. The grand and graceful Chapter-house transformed itself into one of those green bowers, which, once seen, and never to be seen again, make one at once richer and poorer for the rest of life. The fans of groining sprang from the short columns, just as do the feathered boughs of the far more beautiful Maximiliana palm, and just of the same size and shape: and met overhead, as I have seen them meet, in aisles longer by far than our cathedral nave. The free upright shafts, which give such strength, and yet such lightness, to the mullions of each window, pierced upward through those curving lines, as do the stems of young trees through the fronds of palm; and, like them, carried the eye and the fancy up into the infinite, and took off a sense of oppression and captivity which the weight of the roof might have produced. In the nave, in the choir the same vision of the Tropic forest haunted me. The fluted columns not only resembled, but seemed copied from the fluted stems beneath which I had ridden in the primeval woods; their bases, their capitals, seemed copied from the bulgings at the collar of the root, and at the spring of the boughs, produced by a check of the redundant sap; and were garlanded often enough like the capitals of the columns, with delicate tracery of parasite leaves and flowers; the mouldings of the arches seemed copied from the parallel bundles of the curving bamboo shoots; and even the flatter roof of the nave and transepts had its antitype in that highest level of the forest aisles, where the trees, having climbed at last to the light-food which they seek, care no longer to grow upward, but spread out in huge limbs, almost horizontal, reminding the eye of the four-centred arch which marks the period of Perpendicular Gothic.

Nay, to this day there is one point in our cathedral which, to me, keeps up the illusion still. As I enter the choir, and look upward toward the left, I cannot help seeing, in the tabernacle work of the stalls, the slender and aspiring arms of the "rastrajo;" the delicate second growth which, as it were, rushes upward from the earth wherever the forest is cleared; and above it, in the tall lines of the north-west pier of the tower—even though defaced, along the inner face of

the western arch, by ugly and needless perpendicular
panelling—I seem to see the stems of huge Cedars, or
Balatas, or Ceibas, curving over, as they would do, into
the great beams of the transept roof, some seventy feet
above the ground.

Nay, so far will the fancy lead, that I have seemed to
see, in the stained glass between the tracery of the
windows, such gorgeous sheets of colour as sometimes
flash on the eye, when, far aloft, between high stems
and boughs, you catch sight of some great tree ablaze
with flowers, either its own or those of a parasite;
yellow or crimson, white or purple; and over them
again the cloudless blue.

Now, I know well that all these dreams are dreams;
that the men who built our northern cathedrals never
saw these forest forms; and that the likeness of their
work to those of Tropic nature is at most only a corroboration of Mr. Ruskin's dictum, that "the Gothic did
not arise out of, but developed itself into, a resemblance
to vegetation. . . . . It was no chance suggestion of
the form of an arch from the bending of a bough, but
the gradual and continual discovery of a beauty in
natural forms which could be more and more trans-
ferred into those of stone, which influenced at once the
hearts of the people and the form of the edifice." So
true is this, that by a pure and noble copying of the
vegetable beauty which they had seen in their own

clime, the medieval craftsmen went so far—as I have
shown you—as to anticipate forms of vegetable beauty
peculiar to Tropic climes, which they had not seen: a
fresh proof, if proof were needed, that beauty is something absolute and independent of man; and not, as
some think, only relative, and what happens to be
pleasant to the eye of this man or that.

But thinking over this matter, and reading over,
too, that which Mr. Ruskin has written thereon in his
' Stones of Venice,' vol. ii. cap. vi., on the nature of
Gothic, I came to certain further conclusions—or at
least surmises—which I put before you to-night, in
hopes that if they have no other effect on you, they
will at least stir some of you up to read Mr. Ruskin's
works.

Now Mr. Ruskin says, "That the original conception
of Gothic architecture has been derived from vegetation,
from the symmetry of avenues and the interlacing of
branches, is a strange and vain supposition. It is a
theory which never could have existed for a moment in
the mind of any person acquainted with early Gothic:
but, however idle as a theory, it is most valuable as a
testimony to the character of the perfected style."

Doubtless so. But you must remember always that
the subject of my lecture is Grots and Groves; that I
am speaking not of Gothic architecture in general, but
of Gothic ecclesiastical architecture; and more, almost

exclusively of the ecclesiastical architecture of the Teutonic or northern nations; because in them, as I think, the resemblance between the temple and the forest reached the fullest exactness.

Now the original idea of a Christian church was that of a grot; a cave. That is a historic fact. The Christianity which was passed on to us began to worship, hidden and persecuted, in the catacombs of Rome, it may be often around the martyrs' tombs, by the dim light of candle or of torch. The candles on the Roman altars, whatever they have been made to symbolise since then, are the hereditary memorials of that fact. Throughout the North, in these isles as much as in any land, the idea of the grot was, in like wise, the idea of a church. The saint or hermit built himself a cell; dark, massive, intended to exclude light as well as weather; or took refuge in a cave. There he prayed and worshipped, and gathered others to pray and worship round him, during his life. There he, often enough, became an object of worship in his turn, after his death. In after ages his cave was ornamented, like that of the hermit of Montmajour by Arles; or his cell-chapel enlarged, as those of the Scotch and Irish saints have been, again and again; till at last a stately minster rose above it. Still, the idea that the church was to be a grot haunted the minds of builders.

But side by side with the Christian grot there was

throughout the North another form of temple, dedicated to very different gods; namely, the trees from
whose mighty stems hung the heads of the victims of
Odin or of Thor, the horse, the goat, and in time of
calamity or pestilence, of men.   Trees and not grots
were the temples of our forefathers.

Scholars know well—but they must excuse my quoting it for the sake of those who are not scholars—the
famous passage of Tacitus which tells how our forefathers "held it beneath the dignity of the gods to
coop them within walls, or liken them to any human
countenance: but consecrated groves and woods, and
called by the name of gods that mystery which they
held by faith alone;" and the equally famous passage
of Claudian, about "the vast silence of the Black
Forest, and groves awful with ancient superstition;
and oaks, barbarian deities;" and Lucan's "groves
inviolate from all antiquity, and altars stained with
human blood."

To worship in such spots was an abomination to the
early Christian.   It was as much a test of heathendom
as the eating of horse-flesh, sacred to Odin, and therefore unclean to Christian men.   The Lombard laws
and others forbid expressly the lingering remnants of
grove worship.   St. Boniface and other early missionaries hewed down in defiance the sacred oaks, and paid
sometimes for their valour with their lives.

It is no wonder, then, if long centuries elapsed ere
the likeness of vegetable forms began to reappear in
the Christian churches of the North. And yet both
grot and grove were equally the natural temples which
the religious instinct of all deep-hearted peoples, conscious of sin, and conscious, too, of yearnings after a
perfection not to be found on earth, chooses from the
earliest stage of awakening civilisation. In them,
alone, before he had strength and skill to build nobly
for himself, could man find darkness, the mother of
mystery and awe, in which he is reminded perforce of
his own ignorance and weakness; in which he learns
first to remember unseen powers, sometimes to his
comfort and elevation, sometimes only to his terror
and debasement; darkness; and with it silence and
solitude, in which he can collect himself, and shut out
the noise and glare, the meaness and the coarseness, of
the world; and be alone a while with his own thoughts,
his own fancy, his own conscience, his own soul.

But for a while, as I have said, that darkness, solitude, and silence were to be sought in the grot, not in
the grove.

Then Christianity conquered the Empire. It adapted,
not merely its architecture, but its very buildings, to
its worship. The Roman Basilica became the Chris-
tion church; a noble form of building enough, though
one in which was neither darkness, solitude, nor silence,

but crowded congregations, clapping—or otherwise—
the popular preacher; or fighting about the election of
a bishop or a pope, till the holy place ran with Christian blood.   The deep-hearted Northern turned away,
in weariness and disgust, from those vast halls, fitted
only for the feverish superstition of a profligate and
worn-out civilisation; and took himself, amid his own
rocks and forests, moors and shores, to a simpler and
sterner architecture, which should express a creed,
sterner; and at heart far simpler; though dogmatically
the same.

And this is, to my mind, the difference, and the
noble difference, between the so-called Norman architecture, which came hither about the time of the Conquest; and that Romanized Italy.

But the Normans were a conquering race; and one
which conquered, be it always remembered, in England
at least, in the name and by the authority of Rome.
Their ecclesiastics, like the ecclesiastics on the Continent, were the representatives of Roman civilisation, of
Rome's right, intellectual and spiritual, to rule the
world.

Therefore their architecture, like their creed, was
Roman.   They took the massive towering Roman forms,
which expressed domination; and piled them one on
the other, to express the domination of Christian Rome
over the souls, as they had represented the domination

of heathen Rome over the bodies, of men. And so side by side with the towers of the Norman keep rose the towers of the Norman cathedral—the two signs of a double servitude.

But, with the thirteenth century, there dawned an age in Northern Europe, which I may boldly call an heroic age; heroic in its virtues and in its crimes; an age of rich passionate youth, or rather of early manhood; full of aspirations of chivalry, of self-sacrifice as strange and terrible as it was beautiful and noble, even when most misguided. The Teutonic nations of Europe—our own forefathers most of all—having absorbed all that heathen Rome could teach them, at least for the time being, began to think for themselves; to have poets, philosophers, historians, architects, of their own. The thirteenth century was especially an age of aspiration; and its architects expressed, in building, quite unlike those of the preceding centuries, the aspirations of the time.

The Pointed Arch had been introduced half a century before. It may be that the Crusaders saw it in the East and brought it home. It may be that it originated from the quadripartite vaulting of the Normans, the segmental groins of which, crossing diagonally, produced to appearance the pointed arch. It may be that it was derived from that mystical figure of a pointed oval form, the vesica piscis. It may be, lastly, that it was suggested simply by the intersection of semi-circular arches, so frequently found in ornamental arcades. The last cause may perhaps be the true one: but it matters little whence the pointed arch came. It matters much what it meant to those who introduced it. And at the beginning of the Transition or semi-Norman period, it seems to have meant nothing. It was not till the thirteenth century that it had gradually received, as it were, a soul, and had become the exponent of a great idea. As the Norman architecture and its forms had signified domination, so the Early English, as we call it, signified aspiration; an idea which was perfected, as far as it could be, in what we call the Decorated style.

There is an evident gap, I had almost said a gulf, between the architectural mind of the eleventh and that of the thirteenth century. A vertical tendency, a longing after lightness and freedom, appears; and with them a longing to reproduce the graces of nature and art. And here I ask you to look for yourselves at the buildings of this new era—there is a beautiful specimen in yonder arcade *—and judge for yourselves whether they, and even more than they the Decorated style into which they developed, do not remind you of the forest shapes?

And if they remind you: must they not have re-

---

* An arcade in the King's School, Chester.

minded those who shaped them? Can it have been otherwise? We know that the men who built were earnest. The carefulness, the reverence, of their work have given a subject for some of Mr. Ruskin's noblest chapters, a text for some of his noblest sermons. We know that they were students of vegetable form. That is proved by the flowers, the leaves, even the birds, with which they enwreathed their capitals and enriched their mouldings. Look up there, and see.

You cannot look at any good church-work from the thirteenth to the middle of the fifteenth century, without seeing that leaves and flowers were perpetually in the workman's mind. Do you fancy that stems and boughs were never in his mind? He kept, doubtless, in remembrance the fundamental idea, that the Christian church should symbolise a grot or cave. He could do no less; while he again and again saw hermits around him dwelling and worshipping in caves, as they had done ages before in Egypt and Syria; while he fixed, again and again, the site of his convent and his minster in some secluded valley guarded by cliffs and rocks, like Vale Crucis in North Wales. But his minster stood often not among rocks only, but amid trees; in some clearing in the primeval forest, as Vale Crucis was then. At least he could not pass from minster ot minster, from town to town, without journeying through long miles of forest. Do you think that the

x

awful shapes and shadows of that forest never haunted his imagination as he built ? He would have cut down ruthlessly, as his predecessors the early missionaries did, the sacred trees amid which Thor and Odin had been worshipped by the heathen Saxons; amid which still darker deities were still worshipped by the heathen tribes of Eastern Europe. But he was the descendant of men who had worshipped in those groves; and the glamour of them was upon him still. He peopled the wild forest with demons and fairies: but that did not surely prevent his feeling its ennobling grandeur, its chastening loneliness. His ancestors had held the oaks for trees of God, even as the Jews held the Cedar, and the Hindoos likewise; for the Deodara pine is not only, botanists tell us, the same as the Cedar of Lebanon: but its very name—the Deodara—signifies nought else but " The tree of God."

His ancestors, I say, had held the oaks for trees of God. It may be that as the monk sat beneath their shade with his Bible on his knee, like good St. Boniface in the Fulda forest, he found that his ancestors were right.

To understand what sort of trees they were from which he got his inspiration: you must look, not at an average English wood, perpetually thinned out as the trees arrive at middle age. Still less must you look at the pines, oaks, beeches, of an English park, where each tree has had space to develop itself freely into a more or less rounded form. You must not even look at the tropic forests. For there, from the immense diversity of forms, twenty varieties of tree will grow beneath each other, forming a close-packed heap of boughs and leaves, from the ground to a hundred feet and more aloft.

You should look at the North American forests of social trees—especially of pines and firs, where trees of one species, crowded together, and competing with equal advantages for the air and light, form themselves into one wilderness of straight smooth shafts, surmounted by a flat sheet of foliage, held up by boughs like the ribs of a groined roof; while underneath the ground is bare as a cathedral floor.

You all know, surely, the Hemlock spruce of America; which, while growing by itself in open ground, is the most wilful and fantastic, as well as the most graceful, of all the firs; imitating the shape, not of its kindred, but of an enormous tuft of fern.

Yet if you look at the same tree, when it has struggled long for life from its youth amid other trees of its own kind and its own age; you find that the lower boughs have died off from want of light, leaving not a scar behind. The upper boughs have reached at once the light, and their natural term of years. They are content to live, and little more. The central trunk no longer sends up each year a fresh perpendicular shoot to aspire above the rest: but as weary of struggling ambition as they are, is content to become more and more their equal as the years pass by. And this is a law of social forest trees, which you must bear in mind, whenever I speak of the influence of tree-forms on Gothic architecture.

Such forms as these are rare enough in Europe now.

I never understood how possible, how common, they must have been in medieval Europe, till I saw in the forest of Fontainebleau a few oaks like the oak of Charlemagne, and the Bouquet du Roi, at whose age I dare not guess, but whose size and shape showed them to have once formed part of a continuous wood, the like whereof remains not in these isles—perhaps not east of the Carpathian Mountains. In them a clear shaft of at least sixty, it may be eighty feet, carries a flat head of boughs, each in itself a tree. In such a grove, I thought, the heathen Gaul, even the heathen Frank, worshipped, beneath "trees of God." Such trees, I thought, centuries after, inspired the genius of every builder of Gothic aisles and roofs.

Thus, at least, we can explain that rigidity, which Mr. Ruskin tells us, "is a special element of Gothic architecture. Greek and Egyptian buildings," he says —and I should have added, Roman building also, in proportion to their age, *i.e.*, to the amount of the

Roman elements in them—"stand for the most part
by their own weight and mass, one stone passively
incumbent on another: but in the Gothic vaults and
traceries there is a stiffness analogous to that of the
bones of a limb, or fibres of a tree; an elastic tension
and communication of force from part to part; and also
a studious expression of this throughout every part of
the building." In a word, Gothic vaulting and tracery
have been studiously made like to boughs of trees.
Were those boughs present to the mind of the architect? Or is the coincidence merely fortuitous? You
know already how I should answer. The cusped arch,
too, was it actually not intended to imitate vegetation?
Mr. Ruskin seems to think so. He says that it is
merely the special application to the arch of the great
ornamental system of foliation, which, "whether simple
as in the cusped arch, or complicated as in tracery,
arose out of the love of leafage. Not that the form of
the arch is intended to imitate a leaf, but to be invested
with the same characters of beauty which the designer
had discovered in the leaf." Now I differ from Mr.
Ruskin with extreme hesitation. I agree that the
cusped arch is not meant to imitate a leaf. I think
with Mr. Ruskin, that it was probably first adopted on
account of its superior strength; and that it afterwards
took the form of a bough. But I cannot as yet believe
that it was not at last intended to imitate a bough; a

bough of a very common form, and one in which " active rigidity " is peculiarly shown. I mean a bough which has forked. If the lower fork has died off, for want of light, we obtain something like the simply cusped arch. If it be still living—but short and stunted in comparison with the higher fork—we obtain, it seems to me, something like the foliated cusp; both likenesses being near enough to those of common objects to make it possible that those objects may have suggested them. And thus, more and more boldly, the medieval architect learnt to copy boughs, stems, and, at last, the whole effect, as far always as stone would allow, of a combination of rock and tree, of grot and grove.

So he formed his minsters, as I believe, upon the model of those leafy minsters in which he walked to meditate, amid the aisles which God, not man, has built. He sent their columns aloft like the boles of ancient trees. He wreathed their capitals, sometimes their very shafts, with flowers and creeping shoots. He threw their arches out, and interwove the groinings of their vaults, like the bough-roofage overhead. He decked with foliage and fruit the bosses above and the corbels below. He sent up out of those corbels upright shafts along the walls, in the likeness of the trees which sprang. out of the rocks above his head. He raised those walls into great cliffs. He pierced them with the arches of the triforium, as with hermits' cells.

He represented in the horizontal sills of his windows, and in his horizontal string-courses, the horizontal strata of the rocks. He opened the windows into high and lofty glades, broken, as in the forest, by the tracery of stems and boughs, through which was seen, not merely the outer, but the upper world. For he craved, as all true artists crave, for light and colour; and had the sky above been one perpetual blue, he might have been content with it, and left his glass transparent. But in that dark dank northern clime, rain and snow-storm, black cloud and grey mist, were all that he was like to see outside for nine months in the year. So he took such light and colour as nature gave in her few gayer moods; and set aloft his stained glass windows the hues of the noonday and the rainbow, and the sun-rise and the sunset, and the purple of the heather, and the gold of the gorse, and the azure of the bugloss, and the crimson of the poppy; and among them, in gorgeous robes, the angels and the saints of heaven, and the memories of heroic virtues and heroic sufferings, that he might lift up his own eyes and heart for ever out of the dark, dank, sad world of the cold north, with all its coarsenesses and its crimes, toward a realm of perpetual holiness, amid a perpetual summer of beauty and of light; as one who—for he was true to nature, even in that—from between the black jaws of a narrow glen, or from beneath the black shade of gnarled trees, catches a glimpse of far lands gay with gardens and cottages, and purple mountain ranges, and the far-off sea, and the hazy horizon melting into the hazy sky; and finds his heart carried out into an infinite at once of freedom and of repose.

And so out of the cliffs and the forests he shaped the inside of his church. And how did he shape the outside? Look for yourselves, and judge. But look: not at Chester, but at Salisbury. Look at those churches which carry not mere towers, but spires, or at least pinnacled towers approaching the pyramidal form. The outside form of every Gothic cathedral must be considered imperfect if it does not culminate in something pyramidal.

The especial want of all Greek and Roman buildings with which we are acquainted is the absence—save in a few and unimportant cases—of the pyramidal form. The Egyptians knew at least the worth of the obelisk: but the Greeks and Romans hardly knew even that: their buildings are flat-topped. Their builders were contented with the earth as it was. There was a great truth involved in that; which I am the last to deny.

But religions which, like the Buddhist or the Christian, nurse a noble self-discontent, are sure to adopt sooner or later an upward and aspiring form of building. It is not merely that, fancying heaven to be above earth, they point towards heaven. There is a deeper natural language in the pryramidal form of a growing tree. It symbolises growth, or the desire of growth. The Norman tower does nothing of the kind. It does not aspire to grow. Look—I mention an instance with which I am most familiar—at the Norman tower of Bury St. Edmund's. It is graceful—awful, if you will—but there is no aspiration in it.. It is stately : but self-content. Its horizontal courses ; circular arches ; above all, its flat sky-line, seem to have risen enough : and wish to rise no higher. For it has no touch of that unrest of soul, which is expressed by the spire, and still more by the compound spire, with its pinnacles, crockets, finials, which are finials only in name ; for they do not finish, and are really terminal buds, as it were, longing to open and grow upward, even as the crockets are bracts and leaves thrown off as the shoot has grown.

You feel, surely, the truth of these last words. You cannot look at the canopy work or the pinnacle work of this cathedral without seeing that they do not merely suggest buds and leaves, but that the buds and leaves are there carven before your eyes. I myself cannot look at the tabernacle work of our stalls without being reminded of the young pine forests which clothe the Hampshire moors. But if the details are copied from vegetable forms, why not the whole? Is not a spire like a growing tree, a tabernacle like a fir-tree, a

compound spire like a group of firs? And if we can
see that : do you fancy that the man who planned the
spire did not see it as clearly as we do; and perhaps
more clearly still ?

I am aware, of course, that Norman architecture had
sometimes its pinnacle, a mere conical or polygonal
capping. I am aware that this form, only more and
more slender, lasted on in England during the thirteenth and the early part of the fourteenth century;
and on the Continent, under many modifications, one
English kind whereof is usually called a " broach," of
which you have a beautiful specimen in the new church
at Hoole.

Now, no one will deny that that broach is beautiful.
But it would be difficult to prove that its form was
taken from a North European tree. The cypress was
unknown, probably, to our northern architects. The
Lombardy poplar—which has wandered hither, I know
not when, all the way from Cashmere—had not wandered then, I believe, further than North Italy. The
form is rather that of mere stone; of the obelisk, or of
the mountain peak; and they, in fact, may have at
first suggested the spire. The grandeur of an isolated
mountain, even of a dolmen or single upright stone, is
evident to all.

But it is the grandeur, not of aspiration, but of
defiance ; not of the Christian ; not even of the Stoic ;

but rather of the Epicurean. It says—I cannot rise.
I do not care to rise. I will be contentedly and
valiantly that which I am; and face circumstances,
though I cannot conquer them. But it is defiance
under defeat. The mountain-peak does not grow, but
only decays. Fretted by rains, peeled by frost, splintered
by lightning, it must down at last; and crumble into
earth, were it as old, as hard, as lofty as the Matter-
horn itself. And while it stands, it wants not only
aspiration, it wants tenderness; it wants humility; it
wants the unrest which tenderness and humility must
breed, and which Mr. Ruskin so clearly recognises in
the best Gothic art. And, meanwhile, it wants naturalness. The mere smooth spire or broach—I had
almost said, even the spire of Salisbury—is like no tall
or commanding object in Nature. It is merely the
caricature of one; it may be of the mountain-peak.
The outline must be broken, must be softened, before
it can express the soul of a creed which, in the thirteenth and fourteenth centuries far more than now,
was one of penitence as well as of aspiration, of passionate emotion as well as of lofty faith. But a shape
which will express that soul must be sought, not among
mineral, but among vegetable, forms. And remember
always, if we feel thus even now, how much more must
those medieval men of genius have felt thus, whose
work we now dare only copy line by line?

So—as it seems to me—they sought among vegetable forms for what they needed : and they found it at
once in the pine, or rather the fir,—the spruce and silver
firs of their own forests. They are not, of course, indigenous to England. But they are so common through
all the rest of Europe, that not only would the form
suggest itself to a Continental architect, but to any
English clerk who travelled, as all did who could,
across the Alps to Rome. The fir-tree, not growing on
level ground, like the oaks of Fontainebleau, into one
flat roof of foliage, but clinging to the hill-side and
the crag, old above young, spire above spire, whorl
above whorl—for the young shoots of each whorl of
boughs point upward in the spring ; and now and then
a whole bough, breaking away, as it were, into free
space, turns upward altogether, and forms a secondary
spire on the same tree—this surely was the form which
the medieval architect seized, to clothe with it the
sides and roof of the stone mountain which he had
built ; piling up pinnacles and spires, each crocketed
at the angles ; that, like a group of firs upon an isolated
rock, every point of the building might seem in act to
grow toward heaven, till his idea culminated in that
glorious Minster of Cologne, which, if it ever be com-
pleted, will be the likeness of one forest-clothed group
of cliffs, surrounded by three enormous pines.

One feature of the Norman temple he could keep; for

it was copied from the same nature which he was trying to copy—namely, the high-pitched roof and gables. Mr. Ruskin lays it down as a law, that the acute angle in roofs, gables, spires, is the distinguishing mark of northern Gothic. It was adopted, most probably, at first from domestic buildings. A northern house or barn must have a high-pitched roof: or the snow will not slip off it. But that fact was not discovered by man; it was copied by him from the rocks around. He saw the mountain peak jut black and bare above the snows of winter; he saw those snows slip down in sheets, rush down in torrents under the sun, from the steep slabs of rock which coped the hill-side; and he copied, in his roofs, the rocks above his town. But as the love for decorations arose, he would deck his roofs as nature had decked hers, till the grey sheets of the cathedral slates should stand out amid pinnacles and turrets rich with foliage, as the grey mountain sides stood out amid knolls of feathery birch and towering pine.

He failed, though he failed nobly. He never succeeded in attaining a perfectly natural style.

The medieval architects were crippled to the last by the tradition of artificial Roman forms. They began improving them into naturalness, without any clear notion of what they wanted; and when that notion became clear, it was too late. Take, as an instance, the tracery of their windows. It is true, as Mr. Ruskin says, that they began by piercing holes in a wall of the form of a leaf, which developed, in the rose window, into the form of a star inside, and of a flower outside. Look at such aloft there. Then, by introducing mullions and traceries into the lower part of the window, they added stem and bough forms to those flower forms. But the two did not fit. Look at the west window of our choir, and you will see what I mean. The upright mullions break off into bough curves graceful enough : but these are cut short—as I hold, spoiled—by circular and triangular forms of rose and trefoil resting on them as such forms never rest in Nature ; and the whole, though beautiful, is only half beautiful. It is fragmentary, unmeaning, barbaric, because unnatural.

They failed, too, it may be, from the very paucity of the vegetable forms they could find to copy among the flora of this colder clime ; and so, stopped short in drawing from Nature, ran off into mere purposeless luxuriance. Had they been able to add to their stock of memories a hundred forms which they would have seen in the Tropics, they might have gone on for centuries copying Nature without exhausting her.

And yet, did they exhaust even the few forms of beauty which they saw around them ? It must be confessed that they did not. I believe that they could not, because they dared not. The unnaturalness of the creed which they expressed always hampered them. It forbade them to look Nature freely and lovingly in the face. It forbade them—as one glaring example —to know anything truly of the most beautiful of all natural objects—the human form. They were tempted perpetually to take Nature as ornament, not as basis; and they yielded at last to the temptation; till, in the age of Perpendicular architecture, their very ornament became unnatural again; because conventional, untrue, meaningless.

But the creed for which they worked was dying by that time, and therefore the art which expressed it must needs die too. And even that death, or rather the approach of it, was symbolised truly in the flatter roof, the four-centred arch, the flat-topped tower of the fifteenth-century church. The creed had ceased to aspire: so did the architecture. It had ceased to grow: so did the temple. And the arch sank lower; and the rafters grew more horizontal; and the likeness to the old tree, content to grow no more, took the place of the likeness to the young tree struggling toward the sky.

And now—unless you are tired of listening to me— a few practical words.

We are restoring our old cathedral stone by stone after its ancient model. We are also trying to build a new church. We are building it—as most new churches in England are now built—in a pure Gothic style.

Are we doing right? I do not mean morally right. It is always morally right to build a new church, if needed, whatever be its architecture. It is always morally right to restore an old church, if it be beautiful and noble, as an heirloom handed down to us by our ancestors, which we have no right—I say, no right—for the sake of our children, and of our children's children, to leave to ruin.

But are we artistically, æsthetically right? Is the best Gothic fit for our worship? Does it express our belief? Or shall we choose some other style?

I say that it is; and that it is so because it is a style which, if not founded on Nature, has taken into itself more of Nature, of Nature beautiful and healthy, than any other style.

With greater knowledge of Nature, both geographical and scientific, fresh styles of architecture may and will arise, as much more beautiful, and as much more natural, than the Gothic, as Gothic is more beautiful and natural than the Norman. Till then we must take the best models which we have; use them; and, as it were, use them up and exhaust them. By that time we may have learnt to improve on them; and to build churches more Gothic than Gothic itself, more like grot and grove than even a northern cathedral.

That is the direction in which we must work. And if any shall say to us, as it has been said ere now—

"After all, your new Gothic churches are but imitations, shams, borrowed symbols, which to you symbolise nothing. They are Romish churches, meant to express Romish doctrine, built for a Protestant creed which they do not express, and for a Protestant worship which they will not fit." Then we shall answer—Not so. The objection might be true if we built Norman or Romanesque churches; for we should then be returning to that very foreign and unnatural style which Rome taught our forefathers, and from which they escaped gradually into the comparative freedom, the comparative naturalness of that true Gothic of which Mr. Ruskin says so well :—

"It is gladdening to remember that, in its utmost nobleness, the very temper which has been thought most averse to it, the Protestant temper of self-dependence and inquiry, were expressed in every case. Faith and aspiration there were in every Christian ecclesiastical building from the first century to the fifteenth : but the moral habits to which England in this age owes the kind of greatness which she has —the habits of philosophical investigation, of accurate thought, of domestic seclusion and independence, of stern self-reliance, and sincere upright searching into religious truth,—were only traceable in the features which were the distinctive creations of the Gothic schools, in the varied foliage and thorny fretwork, and shadowy niche, and buttressed pier, and fearless height of subtle pinnacle and crested tower, sent 'like an unperplexed question up to heaven.'"

So says Mr. Ruskin. I, for one, endorse his gallant words. And I think that a strong proof of their truth is to be found in two facts, which seem at first paradoxical. First, that the new Roman Catholic churches on the Continent—I speak especially of France, which

Y

is the most highly cultivated Romanist country—are, like those which the Jesuits built in the seventeenth and eighteenth centuries, less and less Gothic. The former were sham-classic; the latter are rather of a new fantastic Romanesque, or rather Byzantinesque style, which is a real retrogression from Gothic towards earlier and less natural schools. Next, that the Puritan communions, the Kirk of Scotland and the English Nonconformists, as they are becoming more cultivated —and there are now many highly cultivated men among them—are introducing Gothic architecture more and more into their churches. There are elements in it, it seems, which do not contradict their Puritanism; elements which they can adapt to their own worship; namely, the very elements which Mr. Ruskin has discerned.

But if they can do so, how much more can we of the Church of England? As long as we go on where our medieval forefathers left off; as long as we keep to the most perfect types of their work, in waiting for the day when we shall be able to surpass them, by making our work even more naturalistic than theirs, more truly expressive of the highest aspirations of humanity: so long we are reverencing them, and that latent Protestantism in them, which produced at last the Reformation.

And if any should say—"Nevertheless, your Protestant Gothic church, though you made it ten times more beautiful, and more symbolic, than Cologne Minster itself, would still be a sham. For where would be your images? And still more, where would be your Host? Do you not know that in the medieval church the vistas of its arcades, the alternations of its lights and shadows, the gradations of its colouring, and all its carefully subordinated wealth of art, pointed to, were concentrated round, one sacred spot, as a curve, however vast its sweep through space, tends at every moment toward a single focus? And that spot, that focus, was, and is still, in every Romish church, the body of God, present upon the altar in the form of bread? Without Him, what is all your building? Your church is empty: your altar bare; a throne without a king; an eye-socket without an eye."

My friends, if we be true children of those old worthies, whom Tacitus saw worshipping beneath the German oaks; we shall have but one answer to that scoff:—

We know it; and we glory in the fact. We glory in it, as the old Jews gloried in it, when the Roman soldiers, bursting through the Temple, and into the Holy of Holies itself, paused in wonder and in awe when they beheld neither God, nor image of God, but —blank yet all-suggestive—the empty mercy-seat.

Like theirs, our altar is an empty throne. For it .

symbolises our worship of Him who dwelleth not in temples made with hands; whom the heaven and the heaven of heavens cannot contain.   Our eye-socket holds no eye.   For it symbolises our worship of that Eye which is over all the earth; which is about our path, and about our bed, and spies out all our ways. We need no artificial and material presence of Deity. For we believe in That One Eternal and Universal Real Presence—of which it is written " He is not far from any one of us; for in God we live, and move, and have our being; " and again, " Lo, I am with you, even to the End of the World; " and again—" Wheresoever two or three are gathered together in My Name, there am I in the midst of them."

He is the God of nature, as well as the God of grace. For ever He looks down on all things which He has made : and behold, they are very good.   And, therefore, we dare offer to Him, in our churches, the most perfect works of naturalistic art, and shape them into copies of whatever beauty He has shown us, in man or woman, in cave or mountain peak, in tree or flower, even in bird or butterfly.

But Himself ?—Who can see Him ?   Except the humble and the contrite heart, to whom He reveals Himself as a Spirit to be worshipped in spirit and in truth, and not in bread, nor wood, nor stone, nor gold, nor quintessential diamond.

So we shall obey the sound instinct of our Christian forefathers, when they shaped their churches into forest aisles, and decked them with the boughs of the woodland, and the flowers of the field : but we shall obey too, that sounder instinct of theirs, which made them at last cast out of their own temples, as misplaced and unnatural things, the idols which they had inherited from Rome.

So we shall obey the sound instinct of our heathen forefathers, when they worshipped the unknown God beneath the oaks of the primeval forests : but we shall obey, too, that sounder instinct of theirs, which taught them this, at least, concerning God—That it was beneath His dignity to coop Him within walls; and that the grandest forms of nature, as well as the deepest consciousness of their own souls, revealed to them a mysterious Being, who was to be beheld by faith alone.

GEORGE BUCHANAN, SCHOLAR.

———•◦•———

THE scholar, in the sixteenth century, was a far more important personage than now. The supply of learned men was very small, the demand for them very great. During the whole of the fifteenth, and a great part of the sixteenth century, the human mind turned more and more from the scholastic philosophy of the Middle Ages to that of the Romans and the Greeks; and found more and more in old Pagan Art an element which Monastic Art had not, and which was yet necessary for the full satisfaction of their craving after the Beautiful. At such a crisis of thought and taste, it was natural that the classical scholar, the man who knew old Rome, and still more old Greece, should usurp the place of the monk, as teacher of mankind; and that scholars should form, for a while, a new and powerful aristocracy, limited and privileged, and all the more redoubtable, because its power lay in intellect, and had been won by intellect alone.

Those who, whether poor or rich, did not fear the

monk and priest, at least feared the "scholar," who held, so the vulgar believed, the keys of that magic lore by which the old necromancers had built cities like Rome, and worked marvels of mechanical and chemical skill, which the degenerate modern could never equal.

If the "scholar" stopped in a town, his hostess probably begged of him a charm against toothache or rheumatism. The penniless knight discoursed with him on alchemy, and the chances of retrieving his fortune by the art of transmuting metals into gold. The queen or bishop worried him in private about casting their nativities, and finding their fates among the stars. But the statesman, who dealt with more practical matters, hired him as an advocate and rhetorician, who could fight his master's enemies with the weapons of Demosthenes and Cicero. Wherever the scholar's steps were turned, he might be master of others, as long as he was master of himself. The complaints which he so often uttered concerning the cruelty of fortune, the fickleness of princes, and so forth, were probably no more just then than such complaints are now. Then, as now, he got his deserts; and the world bought him at his own price. If he chose to sell himself to this patron and to that, he was used and thrown away: if he chose to remain in honourable independence, he was courted and feared.

Among the successful scholars of the sixteenth

century, none surely is more notable than George Buchanan. The poor Scotch widow's son, by force of native wit, and, as I think, by force of native worth, fights his way upward, through poverty and severest persecution, to become the correspondent and friend of the greatest literary celebrities of the Continent, comparable, in their opinion, to the best Latin poets of antiquity; the preceptor of princes; the counsellor and spokesman of Scotch statesmen in the most dangerous of times; and leaves behind him political treatises, which have influenced not only the history of his own country, but that of the civilised world.

Such a success could not be attained without making enemies, perhaps without making mistakes. But the more we study George Buchanan's history, the less we shall be inclined to hunt out his failings, the more inclined to admire his worth. A shrewd, sound-hearted, affectionate man, with a strong love of right and scorn of wrong, and a humour withal which saved him— except on really great occasions—from bitterness, and helped him to laugh where narrower natures would have only snarled,—he is, in many respects, a type of those Lowland Scots, who long preserved his jokes, genuine or reputed, as a common household book.*

---

* So says Dr. Irving, writing in 1817. I have, however, tried in vain to get a sight of this book. I need not tell Scotch scholars how much I am indebted throughout this article to Dr. David Irving's erudite second edition of Buchanan's Life.'

A schoolmaster by profession, and struggling for long years amid the temptations which, in those days, degraded his class into cruel and sordid pedants, he rose from the mere pedagogue to be, in the best sense of the word, a courtier; "One," says Daniel Heinsius, "who seemed not only born for a court, but born to amend it. He brought to his queen that at which she could not wonder enough. For, by affecting a certain liberty in censuring morals, he avoided all offence, under the cloak of simplicity." Of him and his compeers, Turnebus, and Muretus, and their friend Andrea Govea, Ronsard, the French court poet, said that they had nothing of the pedagogue about them but the gown and cap. "Austere in face, and rustic in his looks," says David Buchanan, "but most polished in style and speech; and continually, even in serious conversation, jesting most wittily." "Roughhewn, slovenly, and rude," says Peacham, in his 'Compleat Gentleman,' speaking of him, probably, as he appeared in old age, "in his person, behaviour, and fashion; seldom caring for a better outside than a rugge-gown girt close about him: yet his inside and conceipt in poesie was most rich, and his sweetness and facilitie in verse most excellent." A typical Lowland Scot, as I said just now, he seems to have absorbed all the best culture which France could afford him, without losing the strength, honesty, and humour which he inherited from his Stirlingshire kindred.

The story of his life is easily traced. When an old man, he himself wrote down the main events of it, at the request of his friends; and his sketch has been filled out by commentators, if not always favourable, at least erudite. Born in 1506, at the Moss, in Killearn —where an obelisk to his memory, so one reads, has been erected in this century—of a family "rather ancient than rich," his father dead in the prime of manhood, his grandfather a spendthrift, he and his seven brothers and sisters were brought up by a widowed mother, Agnes Heriot—of whom one wishes to know more; for the rule that great sons have great mothers probably holds good in her case. George gave signs, while at the village school, of future scholarship; and when he was only fourteen, his uncle James sent him to the University of Paris. Those were hard times; and the youths, or rather boys, who meant to become scholars, had a cruel life of it, cast desperately out on the wide world to beg and starve, either into self-restraint and success, or into ruin of body and soul. And a cruel life George had. Within two years he was down in a severe illness, his uncle dead, his supplies stopped; and the boy of sixteen got home, he does not tell how. Then he tried soldiering; and was with Albany's French Auxiliaries at the ineffectual attack on Wark Castle. Marching back through deep snow, he got a fresh illness, which kept him in bed all winter. Then he and his brother were sent to St.

Andrew's, where he got his B.A. at nineteen. The next summer he went to France once more; and "fell," he says, "into the flames of the Lutheran sect, which was then spreading far and wide." Two years of penury followed; and then three years of schoolmastering in the College of St. Barbe, which he has immortalised— at least for the few who care to read modern Latin poetry—in his elegy on 'The Miseries of a Parisian Teacher of the Humanities.' The wretched regent master, pale and suffering, sits up all night preparing his lecture, biting his nails, and thumping his desk; and falls asleep for a few minutes, to start up at the sound of the four o'clock bell, and be in school by five, his Virgil in one hand, and his rod in the other, trying to do work on his own acount at old manuscripts, and bawling all the while at his wretched boys, who cheat him, and pay each other to answer to truants' names. The class is all wrong. "One is barefoot, another's shoe is burst, another cries, another writes home. Then comes the rod, the sound of blows and howls; and the day passes in tears." "Then mass, then another lesson, then more blows; there is hardly time to eat."—I have no space to finish the picture of the stupid misery which, Buchanan says, was ruining his intellect, while it starved his body. However, happier days came. Gilbert Kennedy, Earl of Cassilis, who seems to have been a noble young gentleman, took him as his tutor for

the next five years; and with him he went back to
Scotland.

But there his plain speaking got him, as it did more
than once afterward, into trouble. He took it into his
head to write, in imitation of Dunbar, a Latin poem, in
which St. Francis asks him in a dream to become a
Grey Friar, and Buchanan answered in language which
had the unpleasant fault of being too clever, and—to
judge from contemporary evidence—only too true. The
friars said nothing at first: but when King James
made Buchanan tutor to one of his natural sons, they,
"men professing meekness, took the matter somewhat
more angrily than befitted men so pious in the opinion
of the people." So Buchanan himself puts it: but, to
do the poor friars justice, they must have been angels,
not men, if they did not writhe somewhat under the
scourge which he had laid on them. To be told that
there was hardly a place in heaven for monks, was hard
to hear and bear. They accused him to the king of
heresy: but not being then in favour with James, they
got no answer, and Buchanan was commanded to repeat
the castigation. Having found out that the friars
were not to be touched with impunity, he wrote, he
says, a short and ambiguous poem. But the king,
who loved a joke, demanded something sharp and
stinging, and Buchanan obeyed by writing, but not
publishing, the 'Franciscans,' a long satire, compared

to which the 'Somnium' was bland and merciful. The storm rose. Cardinal Beaton, Buchanan says, wanted to buy him of the king, and then, of course, burn him, as he had just burnt five poor souls: so, knowing James's avarice, he fled to England, through freebooters and pestilence.

There he found, he says, "men of both factions being burned on the same day and in the same fire"—a pardonable exaggeration—" by Henry VIII., in his old age more intent on his own safety than on the purity of religion." So to his beloved France he went again, to find his enemy Beaton ambassador at Paris. The capital was too hot to hold him; and he fled south to Bourdeaux, to Andrea Govea, the Portuguese principal of the College of Guienne. As Professor of Latin at Bourdeaux, we find him presenting a Latin poem to Charles V.; and indulging that fancy of his for Latin poetry which seems to us now-a-days a childish pedantry; which was then—when Latin was the vernacular tongue of all scholars—a serious, if not altogether a useful, pursuit. Of his tragedies, so famous in their day—'the Baptist,' the 'Medea,' the 'Jephtha,' and the 'Alcestis'—there is neither space nor need to speak here, save to notice the bold declamations in the 'Baptist' against tyranny and priestcraft; and to notice also that these tragedies gained for the poor Scotsman, in the eyes of the best scholars of Europe, a credit amounting almost to veneration. When he returned to Paris, he found occupation at once; and—as his Scots biographers love to record—"three of the most learned men in the world taught humanity in the same college," viz., Turnebus, Muretus, and Buchanan.

Then followed a strange episode in his life. A university had been founded at Coimbra, in Portugal, and Andrea Govea had been invited to bring thither what French savans he could collect. Buchanan went to Portugal with his brother Patrick; two more Scotsmen, Dempster and Ramsay: and a goodly company of French scholars, whose names and histories may be read in the erudite pages of Dr. Irving, went likewise. All prospered in the new Temple of the Muses for a year or so. Then its high-priest, Govea, died; and, by a peripeteia too common in those days and countries, Buchanan and two of his friends migrated, unwillingly, from the Temple of the Muses for that of Moloch, and found themselves in the Inquisition.

Buchanan, it seems, had said that St. Augustine was more of a Lutheran than a Catholic on the question of the mass. He and his friends had eaten flesh in Lent; which, he says, almost everyone in Spain did. But he was suspected, and with reason, as a heretic; the Grey Friars formed but one brotherhood throughout Europe; and news among them travelled surely if not fast : so that the story of the satire written in Scotland had reached Portugal. The culprits were imprisoned, examined, bullied—but not tortured—for a year and a half. At the end of that time, the proofs of heresy, it seems, were insufficient; but lest—says Buchanan with honest pride—" they should get the reputation of having vainly tormented a man not altogether unknown," they sent him for some months to a monastery, to be instructed by the monks. " The men," he says, " were neither inhuman nor bad, but utterly ignorant of religion;" and Buchanan solaced himself during the intervals of their instructions, by beginning his Latin translation of the Psalms.

At last he got free, and begged leave to return to France; but in vain. Wearied out at last, he got on board a Candian ship at Lisbon, and escaped to England. But England, he says, during the anarchy of Edward VI.'s reign, was not a land which suited him ; and he returned to his beloved France, to fulfil the hopes which he had expressed in his charming 'Desiderium Lutitiæ,' and the still more charming, because more simple, 'Adventus in Galliam,' in which he bids farewell, in most melodious verse, to " the hungry moors of wretched Portugal, and her clods fertile in naught but penury."

Some seven years succeeded of schoolmastering and verse-writing :—The Latin paraphrase of the Psalms ;

another of tho 'Alcestis' of Euripides; an Epithalamium on the marriage of poor Mary Stuart, noble and sincere, however fantastic and pedantic, after the manner of the times; "Pomps," too, for her wedding, and for other public ceremonies, in which all the heathen gods and goddesses figure; epigrams, panegyrics, satires, much of which latter productions he would have consigned to the dust-heap in his old age, had not his too fond friends persuaded him to republish the follies and coarsenesses of his youth. He was now one of the most famous scholars in Europe, and the intimate friend of all the great literary men. Was he to go on to the end, die, and no more? Was he to sink into the mere pedant; or, if he could not do that, into the mere court versifier?

The wars of religion saved him, as they saved many another noble soul, from that degradation. The events of 1560-1-2 forced Buchanan, as they forced many a learned man besides, to choose whether he would be a child of light or a child of darkness; whether he would be a dilettante classicist, or a preacher—it might be a martyr—of the Gospel. Buchanan may have left France in "the troubles" merely to enjoy in his own country elegant and learned repose. He may have fancied that he had found it, when he saw himself, in spite of his public profession of adherence to the Reformed Kirk, reading Livy every afternoon with his

exquisite young sovereign; master, by her favour, of
the temporalities of Crossraguel Abbey, and by the
favour of Murray, Principal of St. Leonard's College in
St. Andrew's. Perhaps he fancied at times that "to-
morrow was to be as to-day, and much more abundant;"
that thenceforth he might read his folio, and write
his epigram, and joke his joke, as a lazy comfortable
pluralist, taking his morning stroll out to the corner
where poor Wishart had been burned, above the blue
sea and the yellow sands, and looking up to the castle
tower from whence his enemy Beaton's corpse had been
hung out; with the comfortable reflection that quieter
times had come, and that whatever evil deeds Archbishop
Hamilton might dare, he would not dare to put the
Principal of St. Leonard's into the "bottle dungeon."

If such hopes ever crossed Geordie's keen fancy, they
were disappointed suddenly and fearfully. The fire
which had been kindled in France was to reach to
Scotland likewise. "Revolutions are not made with
rose-water;" and the time was at hand when all good
spirits in Scotland, and George Buchanan among them,
had to choose, once and for all, amid danger, confusion,
terror, whether they would serve God or Mammon; for
to serve both would be soon impossible.

Which side, in that war of light and darkness, George
Buchanan took, is notorious. He saw then, as others
have seen since, that the two men in Scotland who

were capable of being her captains in the strife were
Knox and Murray; and to them he gave in his allegiance
heart and soul.

This is the critical epoch in Buchanan's life. By his
conduct to Queen Mary he must stand or fall. It is
my belief that he will stand. It is not my intention
to enter into the details of a matter so painful, so
shocking, so prodigious ; and now that that question is
finally set at rest, by the writings both of Mr. Froude
and Mr. Burton, there is no need to allude to it further,
save where Buchanan's name is concerned. One may
now have every sympathy with Mary Stuart ; one may
regard with awe a figure so stately, so tragic, in one
sense so heroic,—for she reminds one rather of the
heroine of an old Greek tragedy, swept to her doom by
some irresistible fate, than of a being of our own flesh
and blood, and of our modern and Christian times.
One may sympathise with the great womanhood which
charmed so many while she was alive ; which has
charmed, in later years, so many noble spirits who
have believed in her innocence, and have doubtless been
elevated and purified by their devotion to one who
seemed to them an ideal being. So far from regarding her
as a hateful personage, one may feel oneself forbidden to
hate a woman whom God may have loved, and may have
pardoned, to judge from the punishment so swift, and
yet so enduring, which He inflicted. At least, he must

so believe who holds that punishment is a sign of mercy; that the most dreadful of all dooms is impunity. Nay, more, those "casket" letters and sonnets may be a relief to the mind of one who believes in her guilt on other grounds; a relief when one finds in them a tenderness, a sweetness, a delicacy, a magnificent self-sacrifice, however hideously misplaced, which shows what a womanly heart was there; a heart which, joined to that queenly brain, might have made her a blessing and a glory to Scotland, had not the whole character been warped and ruinate from childhood, by an education so abominable, that any one who knows what words she must have heard, what scenes she must have beheld in France, from her youth up, will wonder that she sinned so little : not that she sinned so much. One may feel, in a word, that there is every excuse for those who have asserted Mary's innocence, because their own high-mindedness shrank from believing her guilty: but yet Buchanan, in his own place and time, may have felt as deeply that he could do no otherwise than he did.

The charges against him, as all readers of Scotch literature know well, may be reduced to two heads. 1st. The letters and sonnets were forgeries. Maitland of Lethington may have forged the letters ; Buchanan, according to some, the sonnets. Whoever forged them, Buchanan made use of them in his Detection, knowing them to be forged. 2nd. Whether Mary was innocent or not, Buchanan acted a base and ungrateful part in putting himself in the forefront amongst her accusers. He had been her tutor, her pensioner. She had heaped him with favours; and, after all, she was his queen, and a defenceless woman: and yet he returned her kindness, in the hour of her fall, by invectives fit only for a rancorous and reckless advocate, determined to force a verdict by the basest arts of oratory.

Now as to the "casket" letters. I should have thought they bore in themselves the best evidence of being genuine. I can add nothing to the arguments of Mr. Froude and Mr. Burton, save this: that no one clever enough to be a forger, would have put together documents so incoherent, and so incomplete. For the evidence of guilt which they contain is, after all, slight and indirect, and, moreover, superfluous altogether; seeing that Mary's guilt was open and palpable, before the supposed discovery of the letters, to every person at home and abroad who had any knowledge of the facts. As for the alleged inconsistency of the letters with proven facts: the answer is, that whosoever wrote the letters would be more likely to know facts which were taking place around them than any critic could be one hundred or three hundred years afterwards. But if these mistakes as to facts actually exist in them, they are only a fresh argument for their authenticity. Mary, writing in agony and confusion, might easily make a mistake : forgers would only take too good care to make none.

But the strongest evidence in favour of the letters and sonnets, in spite of the arguments of good Dr. Whittaker and other apologists for Mary, is to be found in their tone. A forger in those coarse days would have made Mary write in some Semiramis or Roxana vein, utterly alien to the tenderness, the delicacy, the pitiful confusion of mind, the conscious weakness, the imploring and most feminine trust which makes the letters, to those who—as I do—believe in them, more pathetic than any fictitious sorrows which poets could invent. More than one touch, indeed, of utter self-abasement, in the second letter, is so unexpected, so subtle, and yet so true to the heart of woman, that —as has been well said—if it was invented there must have existed in Scotland an earlier Shakespeare ; who yet has died without leaving any other sign, for good or evil, of his dramatic genius.

As for the theory (totally unsupported) that Buchanan forged the poem usually called the Sonnets; it is paying old Geordie's genius, however versatile it may have been, too high a compliment to believe that he could have written both them and the Detection ; while it is paying his shrewdness too low a compliment to believe that he could have put into them, out of mere carelessness or stupidity, the well-known line, which seems incompatible with the theory both of the letters and of his own Detection ; and which has ere now been brought forward as a fresh proof of Mary's innocence.

And, as with the letters, so with the sonnets : their delicacy, their grace, their reticene, are so many arguments against their having been forged by any Scot of the sixteenth century, and least of all by one in whose character—whatever his other virtues may have been—delicacy was by no means the strongest point.

As for the complaint that Buchanan was ungrateful to Mary, it must be said : That even if she, and not Murray, had bestowed on him the temporalities of Crossraguel Abbey four years before, it was merely fair pay for services fairly rendered ; and I am not aware that payment, or even favours, however gracious, bind any man's soul and conscience in questions of highest morality and highest public importance.   And the importance of that question cannot be exaggerated.   At a moment when Scotland seemed struggling in death-throes of anarchy, civil and religious, and was in danger of becoming a prey either to England or to France, if there could not be formed out of the heart of her a people, steadfast, trusty, united, strong politically because strong in the fear of God and the desire of righteousness—at such a moment at this, a crime had been committed, the like of which had not been heard in Europe since the tragedy of Joan of Naples. All Europe stood aghast. The honour of the Scottish nation was at stake. More than Mary or Bothwell were known to be implicated in the deed; and—as Buchanan puts it in the opening of his 'De Jure Regni'—"The fault of some few was charged upon all; and the common hatred of a particular person did redound to the whole nation; so that even such as were remote from any suspicion were inflamed by the infamy of men's crimes." *

To vindicate the national honour, and to punish the guilty, as well as to save themselves from utter anarchy, the great majority of the Scotch nation had taken measures against Mary which required explicit justification in the sight of Europe, as Buchanan frankly confesses in the opening of his 'De Jure Regni.' The chief authors of those measures had been summoned, perhaps unwisely and unjustly, to answer for their conduct to the Queen of England. Queen Elizabeth—a fact which was notorious enough then, though it has been forgotten till the last few years—was doing her utmost to shield Mary. Buchanan was deputed, it seems, to speak out for the people of Scotland; and certainly never

---

* From the quaint old translation of 1721, by "A Person of Honour of the Kingdom of Scotland."

people had an abler apologist. If he spoke fiercely, savagely, it must be remembered that he spoke of a fierce and savage matter; if he used—and it may be abused—all the arts of oratory, it must be remembered that he was fighting for the honour, and it may be for the national life, of his country, and striking—as men in such cases have a right to strike—as hard as he could. If he makes no secret of his indignation, and even contempt it must be remembered that indignation and contempt may well have been real with him, while they were real with the soundest part of his countrymen; with that reforming middle class, comparatively untainted by French profligacy, comparatively undebauched by feudal subservience, which has been the leaven which has leavened the whole Scottish people in the last three centuries with the elements of their greatness. If, finally, he heaps up against the unhappy Queen charges which Mr. Burton thinks incredible, it must be remembered that, as he well says, these charges give the popular feeling about Queen Mary; and it must be remembered also, that that popular feeling need not have been altogether unfounded. Stories which are incredible, thank God, in these milder days, were credible enough then, because, alas! they were so often true. Things more ugly than any related of poor Mary, were possible enough—as no one knew better than Buchanan—in that very French court in

which Mary had been brought up; things as ugly were
possible in Scotland then, and for at least a century
later; and while we may hope that Buchanan has
overstated his case, we must not blame him too
severely for yielding to a temptation common to all
men of genius when their creative power is roused to
its highest energy by a great cause and a great indignation.

And that the genius was there, no man can doubt;
one cannot read that "hideously eloquent" description
of Kirk o' Field, which Mr. Burton has well chosen as
a specimen of Buchanan's style, without seeing that we
are face to face with a genius of a very lofty order:
not, indeed, of the loftiest—for there is always in
Buchanan's work, it seems to me, a want of uncon-
sciousness, and a want of tenderness—but still a genius
worthy to be placed beside those ancient writers from
whom he took his manner. Whether or not we agree
with his contemporaries, who say that he equalled
Virgil in Latin poetry, we may place him fairly as a
prose writer by the side of Demosthenes, Cicero, or
Tacitus. And so I pass from this painful subject; only
quoting—if I may be permitted to quote—Mr. Burton's
wise and gentle verdict on the whole. "Buchanan,"
he says, "though a zealous Protestant, had a good deal
of the Catholic and sceptical spirit of Erasmus, and an
admiring eye for everything that was great and beau-

tiful. Like the rest of his countrymen, he bowed himself in presence of the lustre that surrounded the early career of his mistress. More than once he expressed his pride and reverence in the inspiration of a genius deemed by his contemporaries to be worthy of the theme. There is not, perhaps, to be found elsewhere in literature so solemn a memorial of shipwrecked hopes, of a sunny opening and a stormy end, as one finds in turning the leaves of the volume which contains the beautiful epigram 'Nympha Caledoniæ' in one part, the 'Detectio Mariæ Reginæ' in another; and this contrast is, no doubt, a faithful parallel of the reaction in the popular mind. This reaction seems to have been general, and not limited to the Protestant party; for the conditions under which it became almost a part of the creed of the Church of Rome, to believe in her innocence had not arisen."

If Buchanan, as some of his detractors have thought, raised himself by subserviency to the intrigues of the Regent Murray, the best heads in Scotland seem to have been of a different opinion. The murder of Murray did not involve Buchanan's fall. He had avenged it, as far as pen could do it, by that 'Admonition Direct to the Trew Lordis,' in which he showed himself as great a master of Scottish, as he was of Latin prose. His satire of the 'Chameleon,' though its publication was stopped by Maitland, must have been read in manuscript by many of those same "True Lords;" and though there were nobler instincts in Maitland than any Buchanan gave him credit for, the satire breathed an honest indignation against that wily turncoat's misdoings, which could not but rccommend the author to all honest men.   Therefore it was, I presume, and not because he was a rogue, and a hired literary spadassin, that to the best heads in Scotland he seemed so useful, it may be so worthy, a man, that he be provided with continually increasing employment. As tutor to James I.; as director, for a short time, of the chancery; as keeper of the privy seal, and privy councillor; as one of the commissioners for codifying the laws, and again—for in the semi-anarchic state of Scotland, government had to do everything in the way of organisation—in the committee for promulgating a standard Latin grammar; in the committee for reforming the University of St. Andrew's: in all these Buchanan's talents were again and again called for; and always ready.   The value of his work, especially that for the reform of St. Andrew's, must be judged by Scotchmen, rather than by an Englishman: but all that one knows of it justifies Melville's sentence in the well-known passage in his memoirs, wherein he describes the tutors and household of the young King. "Mr. George was a Stoic philosopher, who looked not far before him;" in plain words, a high-minded and

right-minded man, bent on doing the duty which lay
nearest him.   The worst that can be said against him
during these times is, that his name appears with the
sum of £100 against it, as one of those "who were to
be entertained in Scotland by pensions out of England;"
and Ruddiman, of course, comments on the fact by
saying that Buchanan "was at length to act under
the threefold character of malcontent, reformer, and
pensioner:" but it gives no proof whatsoever that
Buchanan ever received any such bribe; and in the very
month, seemingly, in which that list was written—
10th March, 1579—Buchanan had given a proof to the
world that he was not likely to be bribed or bought,
by publishing a book, as offensive probably to Queen
Elizabeth as it was to his own royal pupil; namely, his
famous 'De Jure Regni apud Scotos,' the very primer,
according to many great thinkers, of constitutional
liberty.   He dedicates that book to King James, "not
only as his monitor, but also an importunate and bold
exactor, which in these his tender and flexible years
may conduct him in safety past the rocks of flattery."
He has complimented James already on his abhorrence
of flattery, "his inclination far above his years for
undertaking all heroical and noble attempts, his promp-
titude in obeying his instructors and governors, and all
who give him sound admonition, and his judgment and
diligence in examining affairs, so that no man's autho-

rity can have much weight with him unless it be con-
firmed by probable reasons." Buchanan may have
thought that nine years of his stern rule had eradicated
some of James's ill conditions; the petulance which
made him kill the Master of Mar's sparrow, in trying
to wrest it out of his hand; the carelessness with which
—if the story told by Chytræus, on the authority of
Buchanan's nephew, be true—James signed away his
crown to Buchanan for fifteen days, and only discovered
his mistake by seeing Buchanan act in open court
the character of King of Scots. Buchanan had at last
made him a scholar; he may have fancied that he had
made him likewise a manful man : yet he may have
dreaded that, as James grew up, the old inclinations
would return in stronger and uglier shapes, and that
flattery might be, as it was after all, the cause of
James's moral ruin. He at least will be no flatterer.
He opens the dialogue which he sends to the king,
with a calm but distinct assertion of his mother's
guilt, and a justification of the conduct of men who
were now most of them past helping Buchanan, for
they were laid in their graves ; and then goes on to
argue fairly, but to lay down firmly, in a sort of
Socratic dialogue, those very principles by loyalty to
which the House of Hanover has reigned, and will
reign, over these realms. So with his History of
Scotland ; later antiquarian researches have destroyed

the value of the earlier portions of it : but they have
surely increased the value of those later portions, in
which Buchanan inserted so much which he had
already spoken out in his Detection of Mary.   In that
book also, " liberavit animam suam ; " he spoke his
mind, fearless of consequences, in the face of a king who
he must have known—for Buchanan was no dullard—
regarded him with deep dislike, who might in a few
years be able to work his ruin.

But those few years were not given to Buchanan.
He had all but done his work, and he hastened to get
it over before the night should come wherein no man can
work.   One must be excused for telling—one would
not tell it in a book intended to be read only by
Scotchmen, who know or ought to know the tale already
—how the two Melvilles and Buchanan's nephew
Thomas went to see him in Edinburgh, in September,
1581, hearing that he was ill, and his History still in
the press ; and how they found the old sage, true to
his schoolmaster's instincts, teaching the Hornbook
to his servant-lad ; and how he told them that doing
that was "better than stealing sheep, or sitting idle,
which was as bad," and showed them that dedication
to James I., in which he holds up to his imitation as
a hero whose equal was hardly to be found in history,
that very King David whose liberality to the Romish
Church provoked James's witticism that " David was a

sair saint for the crown." Andrew Melville, so James
Melville says, found fault with the style. Buchanan
replied that he could do no more for thinking of another thing, which was to die. They then went to
Arbuthnot's printing-house, and inspected the history,
as far as that terrible passage concerning Rizzio's burial,
where Mary is represented as " laying the miscreant
almost in the arms of Maud de Valois, the late queen."
Alarmed, and not without reason, at such plain speaking,
they stopped the press, and went back to Buchanan's
house. Buchanan was in bed. " He was going," he
said, " the way of welfare." They asked him to soften
the passage ; the king might prohibit the whole work.
" Tell me, man," said Buchanan, " if I have told the
truth." They could not, or would not, deny it. "Then I
will abide his feud, and all his kin's; pray, pray, to God
for me, and let Him direct all." " So," says Melville,
"before the printing of his chronicle was ended, this most
learned, wise, and godly man ended his mortal life."

Camden has a hearsay story—written, it must be
remembered, in James I.'s time—that Buchanan, on
his death-bed repented of his harsh words against
Queen Mary; and an old Lady Rosyth is said to
have said that when she was young a certain David
Buchanan recollected hearing some such words from
George Buchanan's own mouth. Those who will, may
read what Ruddiman and Love have said, and oversaid,

on both sides of the question : whatever conclusion
they come to, it will probably not be that to which
George Chalmers comes in his life of Ruddiman : that
" Buchanan, like other liars, who by the repetition of
falsehoods are induced to consider the fiction as truth,
had so often dwelt with complacency on the forgeries
of his Detections, and the figments of his History, that
he at length regarded his fictions and his forgeries as
most authentic facts."

At all events his fictions and his forgeries had not
paid him in that coin which base men generally consider the only coin worth having, namely, the good
things of this life.   He left nothing behind him—if at
least Dr. Irving has rightly construed the " Testa-
ment Dative " which he gives in his appendix—save
arrears to the sum of 100*l.* of his Crossraguel pension.
We may believe as we choose the story in Mackenzie's
' Scotch Writers,' that when he felt himself dying, he
asked his servant Young about the state of his funds,
and finding he had not enough to bury himself withal,
ordered what he had to be given to the poor, and said
that if they did not choose to bury him they might let
him lie where he was, or cast him in a ditch, the
matter was very little to him.   He was buried, it
seems, at the expense of the city of Edinburgh, in the
Greyfriars' Churchyard—one says in a plain turf grave
—among the marble monuments which covered the

bones of worse or meaner men ; and whether or not the "Throughstone" which, "sunk under the ground in the Greyfriars," was raised and cleaned by the Council of Edinburgh in 1701, was really George Buchanan's, the reigning powers troubled themselves little for several generations where he lay.

For Buchanan's politics were too advanced for his age. Not only Catholic Scotsmen, like Blackwood, Winzet, and Ninian, but Protestants, like Sir Thomas Craig and Sir John Wemyss, could not stomach the ' De Jure Regni.' They may have had some reason on their side. In the then anarchic state of Scotland, organisation and unity under a common head may have been more important than the assertion of popular rights. Be that as it may, in 1584, only two years after his death, the Scots Parliament condemned his Dialogue and History as untrue, and commanded all possessors of copies to deliver them up, that they might be purged of "the offensive and extraordinary matters" which they contained. The ' De Jure Regni ' was again prohibited in Scotland, in 1664, even in manuscript ; and in 1683, the whole of Buchanan's political works had the honour of being burned by the University of Oxford, in company with those of Milton, Languet, and others, as " pernicious books, and damnable doctrines, destructive to the sacred persons of Princes, their state and government, and of all human

2 A

society." And thus the seed which Buchanan had
sown, and Milton had watered—for the allegation that
Milton borrowed from Buchanan is probably true, and
equally honourable to both—lay trampled into the
earth, and seemingly lifeless, till it tillered out, and
blossomed, and bore fruit to a good purpose, in the
Revolution of 1688.

To Buchanan's clear head and stout heart, Scotland
owes, as England owes likewise, much of her modern
liberty. But Scotland's debt to him, it seems to me,
is even greater on the count of morality, public and
private. What the morality of the Scotch upper
classes was like, in Buchanan's early days, is too
notorious; and there remains proof enough—in the
writings, for instance, of Sir David Lindsay—that the
morality of the populace which looked up to the nobles
as its example and its guide, was not a whit better.
As anarchy increased, immorality was likely to increase
likewise; and Scotland was in serious danger of falling
into such a state as that into which Poland fell, to its
ruin, within a hundred and fifty years after; in which
the savagery of feudalism, without its order or its
chivalry, would be varnished over by a thin coating of
French " civilisation," and, as in the case of Bothwell,
the vices of the court of Paris should be added to those
of the Northern freebooter. To deliver Scotland from
that ruin, it was needed that she should be united into

one people, strong, not in mere political, but in moral
ideas; strong by the clear sense of right and wrong,
by the belief in the government and the judgments of
a living God. And the tone which Buchanan, like
Knox, adopted concerning the great crimes of their
day, helped notably that national salvation. It gathered
together, organised, strengthened, the scattered and
wavering elements of public morality. It assured the
hearts of all men who loved the right and hated the
wrong; and taught a whole nation to call acts by their
just names, whoever might be the doers of them. It
appealed to the common conscience of men. It pro-
claimed a universal and God-given morality, a bar at
which all, from the lowest to the highest, must alike
be judged.

The tone was stern: but there was need of sternness.
Moral life and death were in the balance. If the Scots
people were to be told that the crimes which roused their
indignation were excusable, or beyond punishment, or
to be hushed up and slipped over in any way, there
was an end of morality among them. Every man,
from the greatest to the least, would go and do likewise, according to his powers of evil. That method
was being tried in France, and in Spain likewise,
during those very years. Notorious crimes were hushed
up under pretence of loyalty; excused as political
necessities; smiled away as natural and pardonable

weaknesses. The result was the utter demoralisation, both of France and Spain. Knox and Buchanan, the one from the stand-point of an old Hebrew prophet, the other rather from that of a Juvenal or a Tacitus, tried the other method, and called acts by their just names, appealing alike to conscience and to God. The result was virtue and piety, and that manly independence of soul which is thought compatible with hearty loyalty, in a country labouring under heavy disadvantages, long divided almost into two hostile camps, two rival races.

And the good influence was soon manifest, not only in those who sided with Buchanan and his friends, but in those who most opposed them. The Roman Catholic preachers, who at first asserted Mary's right to impunity, while they allowed her guilt, grew silent for shame, and set themselves to assert her entire innocence; while the Scots who have followed their example have, to their honour, taken up the same ground. They have fought Buchanan on the ground of fact, not on the ground of morality: they have alleged—as they had a fair right to do—the probability of intrigue and forgery in an age so profligate : the improbability that a Queen so gifted by nature and by fortune, and confessedly for a long while so strong and so spotless, should as it were by a sudden insanity have proved so untrue to herself. Their noblest and purest sympa-

thies have been enlisted—and who can blame them ?—
in loyalty to a Queen, chivalry to a woman, pity for
the unfortunate and—as they conceived—the innocent;
but whether they have been right or wrong in their
view of facts, the Scotch partisans of Mary have always
—as far as I know—been right in their view of morals;
they have never deigned to admit Mary's guilt, and
then to palliate it by those sentimental, or rather sensual, theories of human nature, too common in a certain
school of French literature,—too common, alas ! in a
certain school of modern English novels. They have
not said, " She did it; but after all, was the deed so
very inexcusable ?" They have said, " The deed was
inexcusable : but she did not do it." And so the
Scotch admirers of Mary, who have numbered among
them many a pure and noble, as well as many a gifted
spirit, have kept at least themselves unstained; and
have shown, whether consciously or not, that they too
share in that sturdy Scotch moral sense which has
been so much strengthened—as I believe—by the plain
speech of good old George Buchanan.

RONDELET, THE HUGUENOT NATURALIST.*

"APOLLO, god of medicine, exiled from the rest of the earth, was straying once across the Narbonnaise in Gaul, seeking to fix his abode there. Driven from Asia, from Africa, and from the rest of Europe, he wandered through all the towns of the province in search of a place propitious for him and for his disciples. At last he perceived a new city, constructed from the ruins of Maguelonne, of Lattes, and of Substantion. He contemplated long its site, its aspect, its neighbourhood, and resolved to establish on this hill of Montpellier a temple for himself and his priests. All smiled on his desires. By the genius of the soil, by

---

* A Life of Rondelet, by his pupil Laurent Joubert, is to be found appended to his works; and with it an account of his illness and death, by his cousin, Claude Formy, which is well worth the perusal of any man, wise or foolish. Many interesting details beside, I owe to the courtesy of Professor Planchon, of Montpellier, author of a discourse on 'Rondelet et ses Disciples,' which appeared, with a learned and curious Appendice, in the 'Montpellier Médical' for 1866.

the character of the inhabitants, no town is more fit for the culture of letters, and above all of medicine. What site is more delicious and more lovely? A heaven pure and smiling; a city built with magnificence; men born for all the labours of the intellect. All around vast horizons and enchanting sites—meadows, vines, olives, green champaigns; mountains and hills, rivers, brooks, lagoons, and the sea. Everywhere a luxuriant vegetation—everywhere the richest production of the land and the water. Hail to thee, sweet and dear city! Hail, happy abode of Apollo, who spreadest afar the light of the glory of thy name!"

"This fine tirade," says Dr. Maurice Raynaud—from whose charming book on the 'Doctors of the Time of Molière' I quote—"is not, as one might think, the translation of a piece of poetry. It is simply part of a public oration by François Fanchon, one of the most illustrious chancellors of the faculty of medicine of Montpellier in the seventeenth century." "From time immemorial," he says, "'the faculty' of Montpellier had made itself remarkable by a singular mixture of the sacred and the profane. The theses which were sustained there began by an invocation to God, the Blessed Virgin, and St. Luke, and ended by these words:—'This thesis will be sustained in the sacred Temple of Apollo.'"

But however extravagant Chancellor Fanchon's praises

of his native city may seem, they are really not exaggerated. The Narbonnaise, or Languedoc, is perhaps the most charming district of charming France. In the far north-east gleam the white Alps; in the far south-west the white Pyrenees; and from the purple glens and yellow downs of the Cevennes on the north-west, the Herault slopes gently down towards the "Etangs," or great salt-water lagoons, and the vast alluvial flats of the Camargue, the field of Caius Marius, where still run herds of half-wild horses, descended from some ancient Roman stock; while beyond all glitters the blue Mediterranean. The great almond orchards, each one sheet of rose-colour in spring; the mulberry orchards, the oliveyards, the vineyards, cover every foot of available upland soil: save where the ruggid and arid downs are sweet with a thousand odoriferous plants, from which the bees extract the famous white honey of Narbonne. The native flowers and shrubs, of a beauty and richness rather Eastern than European, have made the 'Flora Monspeliensis,' and with it the names of Rondelet and his disciples, famous among botanists; and the strange fish and shells upon its shores afforded Rondelet materials for his immortal work upon the 'Animals of the Sea.' The innumerable wild fowl of the "Bouches du Rhône;" the innumerable songsters and other birds of passage, many of them unknown in these islands, and even in the north of

France itself, which haunt every copse of willow and aspen along the brook sides; the gaudy and curious insects which thrive beneath that clear, fierce, and yet bracing sun-light; all these have made the district of Montpellier a home prepared by Nature for those who study and revere her.

Neither was Chancellor Fanchon misled by patriotism, when he said the pleasant people who inhabit that district are fit for all the labours of the intellect. They are a very mixed race, and like most mixed races, quick-witted, and handsome also. There is probably much Roman blood among them, especially in the towns; for Languedoc, or Gallia Narbonnensis, as it was called of old, was said to be more Roman than Rome itself. The Roman remains are more perfect and more interesting—so the late Dr. Whewell used to say—than any to be seen now in Italy; and the old capital, Narbonne itself, was a complete museum of Roman antiquities ere Francis I. destroyed it, in order to fortify the city upon a modern system against the invading armies of Charles V. There must be much Visigothic blood likewise in Languedoc; for the Visigothic Kings held their courts there from the fifth century, until the time that they were crushed by the invading Moors. Spanish blood, likewise, there may be; for much of Languedoc was held in the early Middle Age by those descendants of Eudes of Acquitaine

who established themselves as kings of Majorca and
Arragon; and Languedoc did not become entirely
French till 1349, when Philip le Bel bought Montpellier of those potentates. The Moors, too, may have
left some traces of their race behind. They held the
country from about A.D. 713 to 758, when they were
finally expelled by Charles Martel and Eudes. One
sees to this day their towers of meagre stone-work,
perched on the grand Roman masonry of those old
amphitheatres, which they turned into fortresses. One
may see, too—so tradition holds—upon those very
amphitheatres the stains of the fires with which Charles
Martel smoked them out; and one may see, too, or fancy
that one sees, in the aquiline features, the bright black
eyes, the lithe and graceful gestures, which are so common in Languedoc, some touch of the old Mahommedan
race, which passed like a flood over that Christian
land.

Whether or not the Moors left behind any traces of
their blood, they left behind, at least, traces of their
learning; for the university of Montpellier claimed to
have been founded by Moors at a date of altogether
abysmal antiquity. They looked upon the Arabian physicians of the Middle Age, on Avicenna and Averrhoes,
as modern innovators, and derived their parentage from
certain mythic doctors of Cordova, who, when the Moors
were expelled from Spain in the eighth century, fled to

Montpellier, bringing with them traditions of that primeval science which had been revealed to Adam while still in Paradise; and founded Montpellier, the mother of all the universities in Europe. Nay, some went further still, and told of Bengessaus and Ferragius, the physicians of Charlemagne, and of Marilephus, chief physician of King Chilperic, and even—if a letter of St. Bernard's was to be believed—of a certain bishop who went as early as the second century to consult the doctors of Montpellier; and it would have been in vain to reply to them that in those days, and long after them, Montpellier was not yet built. The facts are said to be: that as early as the beginning of the thirteenth century Montpellier had its schools of law, medicine, and arts, which were erected into a university by Pope Nicholas IV. in 1289.

The university of Montpellier, like—I believe—most foreign ones, resembled more a Scotch than an English university. The students lived, for the most part, not in colleges, but in private lodgings, and constituted a republic of their own, ruled by an abbé of the scholars, one of themselves, chosen by universal suffrage. A terror they were often to the respectable burghers, for they had all the right to carry arms; and a plague likewise, for, if they ran in debt, their creditors were forbidden to seize their books, which, with their swords, were generally all the property they possessed. If, moreover, any one set up a noisy or unpleasant trade near their lodgings, the scholars could compel the town authorities to turn him out. They were most of them, probably, mere boys of from twelve to twenty, living poorly, working hard, and—those at least of them who were in the colleges—cruelly beaten daily, after the fashion of those times; but they seem to have comforted themselves under their troubles by a good deal of wild life out of school, by rambling into the country on the festivals of the saints, and now and then by acting plays; notably, that famous one which Rabelais wrote for them in 1531: " The moral comedy of the man who had a dumb wife;" which "joyous patclinago" remains unto this day in the shape of a well-known comic song. That comedy young Rondelet must have seen acted. The son of a druggist, spicer, and grocer— the three trades were then combined—in Montpellier, and born in 1507, he had been destined for the cloister, being a sickly lad. His uncle, one of the canons of Maguelonne, near by, had even given him the revenues of a small chapel—a job of nepotism which was common enough in those days. But his heart was in science and medicine. He set off, still a mere boy, to Paris to study there; and returned to Montpellier, at the age of eighteen, to study again.

The next year, 1530, while still a scholar himself, he was appointed procurator of the scholars—a post which

brought him in a small fee on each matriculation—and
that year he took a fee, among others, from one of the
most remarkable men of that or of any age, François
Rabelais himself.

And what shall I say of him ?—who stands alone,
like Shakespeare, in his generation; possessed of colossal
learning—of all science which could be gathered in
his days—of practical and statesmanlike wisdom—of
knowledge of languages, ancient and modern, beyond
all his compeers—of eloquence, which when he speaks
of pure and noble things becomes heroic, and, as it
were, inspired—of scorn for meanness, hypocrisy, ignorance—of esteem, genuine and earnest, for the Holy
Scriptures, and for the more moderate of the Reformers
who were spreading the Scriptures in Europe,—and all
this great light wilfully hidden, not under a bushel,
but under a dunghill. He is somewhat like Socrates in
face, and in character likewise ; in him, as in Socrates,
the demigod and the satyr, the man and the ape, are
struggling for the mastery. In Socrates, the true man
conquers, and comes forth high and pure ; in Rabelais’
alas! the victor is the ape, while the man himself sinks
down in cynicism, sensuality, practical jokes, foul talk.
He returns to Paris, to live an idle, luxurious life ; to
die—says the legend—saying, " I go to seek a great
perhaps," and to leave behind him little save a school of
Pantagruelists—careless young gentlemen, whose ideal

was to laugh at everything, to believe in nothing, and to gratify their five senses like the brutes which perish. There are those who read his books to make them laugh; the wise man, when he reads them, will be far more inclined to weep. Let any young man who may see these words remember, that in him, as in Rabelais, the ape and the man are struggling for the mastery. Let him take warning by the fate of one who was to him as a giant to a pigmy; and think of Tennyson's words:—

> "Arise, and fly
> The reeling faun, the sensual feast;
> Strive upwards, working out the beast,
> And let the ape and tiger die."

But to return. Down among them there at Montpellier, like a brilliant meteor, flashed this wonderful Rabelais, in the year 1530. He had fled, some say, for his life. Like Erasmus, he had no mind to be a martyr, and he had been terrified at the execution of poor Louis de Berquin, his friend, and the friend of Erasmus likewise. This Louis de Berquin, a man well known in those days, was a gallant young gentleman and scholar, holding a place in the court of Francis I., who had translated into French the works of Erasmus, Luther, and Melancthon, and had asserted that it was heretical to invoke the Virgin Mary instead of the Holy Spirit, or to call her our Hope and our Life, which titles— Berquin averred—belonged alone to God. Twice had

the doctors of the Sorbonne, with that terrible per-
secutor, Noel Beda, at their head, seized poor Berquin,
and tried to burn his books and him; twice had that
angel in human form, Marguerite d'Angoulême, sister
of Francis I., saved him from their clutches; but when
Francis—taken prisoner at the battle of Pavia—at last
returned from his captivity in Spain, the suppression
of heresy and the burning of heretics seemed to him
and to his mother, Louise of Savoy, a thank-offering
so acceptable to God, that Louis Berquin—who would
not, in spite of the entreaties of Erasmus, purchase his
life by silence—was burnt at last on the Place de Grève,
being first strangled, because he was of gentle blood.

Montpellier received its famous guest joyfully. Rabelais was now forty-two years old, and a distinguished
savant; so they excused him his three years' undergraduate's career, and invested him at once with the
red gown of the bachelors. That red gown—or, rather,
the ragged phantom of it—is still shown at Montpellier,
and must be worn by each bachelor when he takes his
degree. Unfortunately, antiquarians assure us that
the precious garment has been renewed again and again
—the students having clipped bits of it away for relics,
and clipped as earnestly from the new gowns as their
predecessors had done from the authentic original.

Doubtless, the coming of such a man among them to
lecture on the Aphorisms of Hippocrates, and the Ars

Parva of Galen, not from the Latin translations then in use, but from original Greek texts, with comments and corrections of his own, must have had a great influence on the minds of the Montpellier students; and still more influence—and that not altogether a good one —must Rabelais' lighter talk have had, as he lounged— so the story goes—in his dressing-gown upon the public place, picking up quaint stories from the cattle-drivers off the Cevennes, and the villagers who came in to sell their olives and their grapes, their vinegar and their vine-twig faggots, as they do unto this day. To him may be owing much of the sound respect for natural science, and much, too, of the contempt for the super- stition around them, which is notable in that group of great naturalists who were boys in Montpellier at that day. Rabelais seems to have liked Rondelet, and no wonder : he was a cheery, lovable, honest little fellow, very fond of jokes, a great musician and player on the violin, and who, when he grew rich, liked nothing so well as to bring into his house any buffoon or strolling player to make fun for him. Vivacious he was, hot- tempered, forgiving, and with a power of learning and a power of work which were prodigious, even in those hard-working days. Rabelais chaffs Rondelet, under the name of Rondibilis ; for, indeed, Rondelet grew up into a very round, fat, little man ; but Rabelais puts excellent sense into his mouth, cynical enough, and too cynical, but both learned and humorous ; and, if he laughs at him for being shocked at the offer of a fee, and taking it, nevertheless, kindly enough, Rondelet is not the first doctor who has done that, neither will he be the last.

Rondelet, in his turn, put on the red robe of the bachelor, and received, on taking his degree, his due share of fisticuffs from his dearest friends, according to the ancient custom of the University of Montpellier. He then went off to practise medicine in a village at the foot of the Alps, and, half-starved, to teach little children. Then he found he must learn Greek ; went off to Paris a second time, and alleviated his poverty there somewhat by becoming tutor to a son of the Viscomte de Turenne. There he met Gonthier of Andernach, who had taught anatomy at Louvain to the great Vesalius, and learned from him to dissect. We next find him setting up as a medical man amid the wild volcanic hills of the Auvergne, struggling still with poverty, like Erasmus, like George Buchanan, like almost every great scholar in those days ; for students then had to wander from place to place, generally on foot, in search of new teachers, in search of books, in search of the necessaries of life ; undergoing such an amount of bodily and mental toil as makes it wonderful that all of them did not—as some of them doubtless did—die under the hard

2 B

training, or, at best, desert the penurious Muses for the paternal shop or plough.

Rondelet got his doctorate in 1537, and next year fell in love with and married a beautiful young girl called Jeanne Sandre, who seems to have been as poor as he.

But he had gained, meanwhile, a powerful patron; and the patronage of the great was then as necessary to men of letters as the patronage of the public is now. Guillaume Pellicier, Bishop of Maguelonne—or rather then of Montpellier itself, whither he had persuaded Paul II. to transfer the ancient see—was a model of the literary gentleman of the sixteenth century; a savant, a diplomat, a collector of books and manuscripts, Greek, Hebrew, and Syriac, which formed the original nucleus of the present library of the Louvre; a botanist, too, who loved to wander with Rondelet collecting plants and flowers. He retired from public life to peace and science at Montpellier, when to the evil days of his master, Francis I., succeeded the still worse days of Henry II., and Diana of Poitiers. That Jezebel of France could conceive no more natural or easy way of atoning for her own sins than that of hunting down heretics, and feasting her wicked eyes —so it is said—upon their dying torments. Bishop Pellicier fell under suspicion of heresy: very probably with some justice. He fell, too, under suspicion of leading a life unworthy of a celibate churchman, a fault which—if it really existed—was, in those days, pardonable enough in an orthodox prelate, but not so in one whose orthodoxy was suspected. And for a while Pellicier was in prison. After his release he gave himself up to science, with Rondelet and the school of disciples who were growing up around him. They rediscovered together the Garum, that classic sauce, whose praises had been sung of old by Horace, Martial, and Ausonius; and so childlike, superstitious if you will, was the reverence in the sixteenth century for classic antiquity, that when Pellicier and Rondelet discovered that the Garum was made from the fish called Picarel—called Garon by the fishers of Antibes, and Giroli at Venice, both these last names corruptions of the Latin Gerres—then did the two fashionable poets of France, Etienne Dolet and Clement Marot, think it not unworthy of their muse to sing the praises of the sauce which Horace had sung of old. A proud day, too, was it for Pellicier and Rondelet, when wandering somewhere in the marshes of the Camargue, a scent of garlic caught the nostrils of the gentle bishop, and in the lovely pink flowers of the water-germander he recognised the Scordium of the ancients. "The discovery," says Professor Planchon, "made almost as much noise as that of the famous Garum; for at that moment of naïve fervour on behalf of antiquity, to rediscover a plant of Dioscorides or of Pliny was a good fortune and almost an event."

I know not whether, after his death, the good bishop's bones reposed beneath some gorgeous tomb, bedizened with the incongruous half-Pagan statues of the Renaissance: but this, at least, is certain, that Rondelet's disciples imagined for him a monument more enduring than of marble or of brass, more graceful and more curiously wrought than all the sculptures of Torrigiano or Cellini, Baccio Bandinelli or Michael Angelo himself. For they named a lovely little lilac snapdragon, *Linaria Domini Pellicerii,*—" Lord Pellicier's toad-flax ; " and that name it will keep, we may believe, as long as winter and summer shall endure.

But to return. To this good patron—who was the Ambassador at Venice—the newly-married Rondelet determined to apply for employment ; and to Venice he would have gone, leaving his bride behind, had he not been stayed by one of those angels who sometimes walk the earth in women's shape. Jeanne Sandre had an elder sister, Catherine, who had brought her up. She was married to a wealthy man, but she had no children of her own. For four years she and her good husband had let the Rondelets lodge with them, and now she was a widow, and to part with them was more than she could bear. She carried Rondelet off from the students who were seeing him safe out of the city, brought him back, settled on him the same day half her fortune, and soon after settled on him the whole, on the sole condition that she should live with him and her sister. For years afterwards she watched over the pretty young wife and her two girls and three boys—the three boys, alas! all died young—and over Rondelet himself, who, immersed in books and experiments, was utterly careless about money; and was to them all a mother, advising, guiding, managing, and regarded by Rondelet with genuine gratitude as his guardian angel.

Honour and good fortune, in the worldly sense, now poured in upon the druggist's son. Pellicier, his own bishop, stood godfather to his first-born daughter. Montluc, Bishop of Valence, and that wise and learned statesman, the Cardinal of Tournon, stood godfathers a few years later to his twin boys; and what was of still more solid worth to him, Cardinal Tournon took him to Antwerp, Bordeaux, Bayonne, and more than once to Rome; and in these Italian journeys of his he collected many facts for the great work of his life, that 'History of Fishes' which he dedicated, naturally enough, to the cardinal. This book with its plates is, for the time, a masterpiece of accuracy. Those who are best acquainted with the subject say, that it is up to the present day a key to the whole ichthyology of the Mediterranean. Two other men, Belon and Salviani, were then at work

on the same subject, and published their books almost
at the same time ; a circumstance which caused, as was
natural, a three-cornered duel between the supporters
of the three naturalists, each party accusing the other
of plagiarism. The simple fact seems to be that the
almost simultaneous appearance of the three books
in 1554-5 is one of those coincidences inevitable at
moments when many minds are stirred in the same
direction by the same great thoughts—coincidences
which have happened in our own day on questions of
geology, biology, and astronomy ; and which, when the
facts have been carefully examined, and the first flush
of natural jealousy has cooled down, have proved only
that there were more wise men than one in the world
at the same time.

And this sixteenth century was an age in which the
minds of men were suddenly and strangely turned to
examine the wonders of nature with an earnestness,
with a reverence, and therefore with an accuracy,
with which they had never been investigated before.
"Nature," says Professor Planchon, "long veiled in
mysticism and scholasticism, was opening up infinite
vistas. A new superstition, the exaggerated worship
of the ancients, was nearly hindering this movement
of thought towards facts. Nevertheless learning did
her work. She rediscovered, reconstructed, purified,
commented on the texts of ancient authors. Then

came in observation, which showed that more was to be seen in one blade of grass than in any page of Pliny. Rondelet was in the middle of this crisis a man of transition, while he was one of progress. He reflected the past; he opened and prepared the future. If he commented on Dioscorides, if he remained faithful to the theories of Galen, he founded in his 'History of Fishes' a monument which our century respects. He is above all an inspirer, an initiator; and if he wants one mark of the leader of a school, the foundation of certain scientific doctrines, there is in his speech what is better than all systems, the communicative power which urges a generation of disciples along the path of independent research, with Reason for guide, and Faith for aim."

Around Rondelet, in those years, sometimes indeed in his house—for professors in those days took private pupils as lodgers—worked the group of botanists whom Linnæus calls "the Fathers," the authors of the descriptive botany of the sixteenth century. Their names, and those of their disciples and their disciples again, are household words in the mouth of every gardener, immortalised, like good Bishop Pellicier, in the plants which have been named after them. The Lobelia commemorates Lobel, one of Rondelet's most famous pupils, who wrote those 'Adversaria' which contain so many curious sketches of Rondelet's botanical expeditions, and who inherited his botanical (as Joubert his biographer inherited his anatomical) manuscripts. The Magnolia commemorates the Magnols; the Sarracenia, Sarrasin of Lyons; the Bauhinia, Jean Bauhin; the Fuchsia, Bauhin's earlier German master, Leonard Fuchs; and the Clusia—the received name of that terrible "Matapalo," or "Scotch attorney," of the West Indies, which kills the hugest tree, to become as huge a tree itself—immortalizes the great Clusius, Charles de l'Escluse, citizen of Arras, who after studying civil law at Louvain, philosophy at Marburg, and theology at Wittemberg under Melancthon, came to Montpellier in 1551, to live in Rondelet's own house, and become the greatest botanist of his age.

These were Rondelet's palmy days. He had got a theatre of anatomy built at Montpellier, where he himself dissected publicly. He had, says tradition, a little botanic garden, such as were springing up then in several universities, specially in Italy. He had a villa outside the city, whose tower, near the modern railway station, still bears the name of the "Mas de Rondelet." There, too, may be seen the remnants of the great tanks, fed with water brought through earthen pipes from the Fountain of Albe, wherein he kept the fish whose habits he observed. Professor Planchon thinks that he had salt-water tanks likewise; and thus he may have been the father of all "Aquariums." He had a

large and handsome house in the city itself, a large practice as physician in the country round; money flowed
in fast to him, and flowed out fast likewise. He spent
much upon building, pulling down, rebuilding, and
sent the bills in seemingly to his wife and to his guardian angel Catherine. He himself had never a penny
in his purse: but earned the money, and let his ladies
spend it; an equitable and pleasant division of labour
which most married men would do well to imitate. A
generous, affectionate, careless little man, he gave
away, says his pupil and biographer, Joubert, his
valuable specimens to any savant who begged for
them, or left them about to be stolen by visitors, who,
like too many collectors in all ages, possessed light
fingers and lighter consciences. So pacific was he
meanwhile, and so brave withal, that even in the
fearful years of the troubles, he would never carry
sword, nor even tuck or dagger; but went about on
the most lonesome journeys as one who wore a charmed
life, secure in God and in his calling, which was to
heal, and not to kill.

These were the golden years of Rondelet's life; but
trouble was coming on him, and a stormy sunset after
a brilliant day. He lost his sister-in-law, to whom he
owed all his fortunes, and who had watched ever since
over him and his wife like a mother; then he lost his
wife herself under most painful circumstances; then

his best-beloved daughter. Then he married again, and lost the son who was born to him; and then came, as to many of the best in those days, even sorer trials, trials of the conscience, trials of faith.

For in the mean time Rondelet had become a Protestant, like many of the wisest men round him; like, so it would seem from the event, the majority of the university and the burghers of Montpellier. It is not to be wondered at. Montpellier was a sort of half-way resting-place for Protestant preachers, whether fugitive or not, who were passing from Basle, Geneva, or Lyons, to Marguerite of Navarre's little Protestant court at Pau or at Nerac, where all wise and good men, and now and then some foolish and fanatical ones, found shelter and hospitality. Thither Calvin himself had been, passing probably through Montpellier, and leaving —as such a man was sure to leave—the mark of his foot behind him. At Lyons, no great distance up the Rhone, Marguerite had helped to establish an organised Protestant community; and when in 1536 she herself had passed through Montpellier, to visit her brother at Valence, and Montmorency's camp at Avignon, she took with her doubtless Protestant chaplains of her own, who spoke wise words—it may be that she spoke wise words herself—to the ardent and inquiring students of Montpellier. Moreover, Rondelet and his disciples had been for years past in constant communication with the Protestant savants of Switzerland and Germany, among whom the knowledge of nature was progressing as it never had progressed before. For—it is a fact always to be remembered—it was only in the free air of Protestant countries the natural sciences could grow and thrive. They sprung up, indeed, in Italy after the restoration of Greek literature in the fifteenth century; but they withered there again only too soon under the blighting upas shade of superstition. Transplanted to the free air of Switzerland, of Germany, of Britain, and of Montpellier, then half Protestant, they developed rapidly and surely, simply because the air was free; to be checked again in France by the return of superstition with despotism superadded, until the eve of the great French Revolution.

So Rondelet had been for some years Protestant. He had hidden in his house for a long while a monk who had left his monastery. He had himself written theological treatises : but when his Bishop Pellicier was imprisoned on a charge of heresy, Rondelet burnt his manuscripts, and kept his opinions to himself. Still he was a suspected heretic, at last seemingly a notorious one; for only the year before his death, going to visit patients at Perpignan, he was waylaid by the Spaniards, and had to get home through by-passes of the Pyrenees, to avoid being thrown into the Inquisition.

And those were times in which it was necessary for a man to be careful, unless he had made up his mind to be burned. For more than thirty years of Rondelet's life the burning had gone on in his neighbourhood; intermittently it is true: the spasms of superstitious fury being succeeded, one may charitably hope, by pity and remorse: but still the burnings had gone on. The Benedictine monk of St. Maur, who writes the history of Languedoc, says, quite *en passant*, how some one was burnt at Toulouse in 1553, luckily only in effigy, for he had escaped to Geneva: but he adds, " next year they burned several heretics," it being not worth while to mention their names. In 1556 they burned alive at Toulouse Jean Escalle, a poor Franciscan monk, who had found his order intolerable; while one Pierre de Lavaur, who dared preach Calvinism in the streets of Nismes, was hanged and burnt. So had the score of judicial murders been increasing year by year, till it had to be, as all evil scores have to be in this world, paid off with interest, and paid off especially against the ignorant and fanatic monks who for a whole generation, in every university and school in France, had been howling down sound science, as well as sound religion; and at Montpellier in 1560-1, their debt was paid them in a very ugly way. News came down to the hot southerners of Languedoc of the so-called conspiracy of Amboise.—How the Duc de Guise and the

Cardinal de Lorraine had butchered the best blood in France under the pretence of a treasonable plot; how the King of Navarre and the Prince de Condé had been arrested; then how Condé and Coligny were ready to take up arms at the head of all the Huguenots of France, and try to stop this life-long torturing, by sharp shot and cold steel; then how in six months' time the king would assemble a general council to settle the question between Catholics and Huguenots. The Huguenots, guessing how that would end, resolved to settle the question for themselves. They rose in one city after another, sacked the churches, destroyed the images, put down by main force superstitious processions and dances; and did many things only to be excused by the exasperation caused by thirty years of cruelty. At Montpellier there was hard fighting, murders—so say the Catholic historians—of priests and monks, sack of the new cathedral, destruction of the noble convents which lay in a ring round Montpellier. The city and the university were in the hands of the Huguenots, and Montpellier became Protestant on the spot.

Next year came the counter blow. There were heavy battles with the Catholics all round the neighbourhood, destruction of the suburbs, threatened siege and sack, and years of misery and poverty for Montpellier and all who were therein.

Horrible was the state of France in those times of the wars of religion which began in 1562; the times which are spoken of usually as "The Troubles," as if men did not wish to allude to them too openly. Then, and afterwards in the wars of the League, deeds were done for which language has no name. The population decreased. The land lay untilled. The fair face of France was blackened with burnt homesteads and ruined towns. Ghastly corpses dangled in rows upon the trees, or floated down the blood-stained streams. Law and order were at an end. Bands of robbers prowled in open day, and bands of wolves likewise. But all through the horrors of the troubles we catch sight of the little fat doctor riding all unarmed to see his patients throughout Languedoc; going vast distances, his biographers say, by means of regular relays of horses, till he too broke down. Well for him, perhaps, that he broke down when he did; for capture and recapture, massacre and pestilence, were the fate of Montpellier and the surrounding country, till the better times of Henry IV. and the Edict of Nantes in 1598, when liberty of worship was given to the Protestants for a while.

In the burning summer of 1566 Rondeletius went a long journey to Toulouse, seemingly upon an errand of charity, to settle some law affairs for his relations. The sanitary state of the southern cities is bad enough still. It must have been horrible in those days of barbarism and misrule. Dysentery was epidemic at Toulouse then, and Rondelet took it. He knew from the first that he should die. He was worn out, it is said, by over-exertion ; by sorrow for the miseries of the land ; by fruitless struggles to keep the peace, and to strive for moderation in days when men were all immoderate. But he rode away a day's journey—he took two days over it, so weak he was—in the blazing July sun, to a friend's sick wife at Realmont, and there took to his bed, and died a good man's death. The details of his death and last illness were written and published by his cousin Claude Formy ; and well worth reading they are to any man who wishes to know how to die. Rondelet would have no tidings of his illness sent to Montpellier. He was happy, he said, in dying away from the tears of his household, and " safe from insult." He dreaded, one may suppose, lest priests and friars should force their way to his bedside, and try to extort some recantation from the great savant, the honour and glory of their city. So they sent for no priest to Realmont : but round his bed a knot of Calvinist gentlemen and ministers read the Scriptures, and sang David's psalms, and prayed ; and Rondelet prayed with them through long agonies, and so went home to God.

The Benedictine monk-historian of Languedoc, in all

his voluminous folios, never mentions, as far as I can find, Rondelet's existence. Why should he? The man was only a druggist's son and a heretic, who healed diseases, and collected plants, and wrote a book on fish. But the learned men of Montpellier, and of all Europe, had a very different opinion of him. His body was buried at Realmont: but before the schools of Toulouse they set up a white marble slab, and an inscription thereon setting forth his learning and his virtues; and epitaphs on him were composed by the learned throughout Europe, not only in French and Latin, but in Greek, Hebrew, and even Chaldee.

So lived and so died a noble man; more noble—to my mind—than many a victorious warrior, or successful statesman, or canonised saint. To know facts, and to heal diseases, were the two objects of his life. For them he toiled, as few men have toiled; and he died in harness, at his work—the best death any man can die.

VESALIUS THE ANATOMIST.

I cannot begin a sketch of the life of this great man better than by trying to describe a scene so pictu- resque, so tragic in the eyes of those who are wont to mourn over human follies, so comic in the eyes of those who prefer to laugh over them, that the reader will not be likely to forget either it or the actors in it.

It is a darkened chamber in the College of Alcala, in the year 1562, where lies, probably in a huge four-post bed, shrouded in stifling hangings, the heir-apparent of the greatest empire in the then world, Don Carlos, only son of Philip II., and heir-apparent of Spain, the Netherlands, and all the Indies. A short sickly boy of sixteen, with a bull head, a crooked shoulder, a short leg, and a brutal temper, he will not be missed by the world if he should die. His profligate career seems to have brought its own punishment. To the scandal of his father, who tolerated no one's vices save his own,

2 o

as well as to the scandal of the university authorities
of Alcala, he has been scouring the streets at the head
of the most profligate students, insulting women, even
ladies of rank, and amenable only to his lovely young
stepmother, Elizabeth of Valois, Isabel de la Paz, as
the Spaniards call her, the daughter of Catherine de
Medicis, and sister of the King of France. Don Carlos
should have married her, had not his worthy father
found it more advantageous for the crown of Spain, as
well as more pleasant for him, Philip, to marry her
himself. Whence came heart-burnings, rage, jealousies,
romances, calumnies, of which two last—in as far at
least as they concern poor Elizabeth—no wise man
now believes a word.

Going on some errand on which he had no business
—there are two stories, neither of them creditable nor
necessary to repeat—Don Carlos has fallen down stairs
and broken his head. He comes, by his Portuguese
mother's side, of a house deeply tainted with insanity ;
and such an injury may have serious consequences.
However, for nine days the wound goes on well, and
Don Carlos, having had a wholesome fright, is
according to Doctor Olivarez, the *medico de camara,*
a very good lad, and lives on chicken broth and dried
plums. But on the tenth day comes on numbness of
the left side, acute pains in the head, and then
gradually shivering, high fever, erysipelas. His head

and neck swell to an enormous size; then comes raging delirium, then stupefaction, and Don Carlos lies as one dead.

A modern surgeon would, probably, thanks to that training of which Vesalius may be almost called the father, have had little difficulty in finding out what was the matter with the luckless lad, and little difficulty in removing the evil, if it had not gone too far. But the Spanish physicians were then, as many of them are said to be still, as far behind the world in surgery as in other things; and indeed surgery itself was then in its infancy, because men, ever since the early Greek schools of Alexandria had died out, had been for centuries feeding their minds with anything rather than with facts. Therefore the learned morosophs who were gathered round Don Carlos's sick bed had become, according to their own confession, utterly confused, terrified, and at their wits' end.

It is the 7th of May, the eighteenth day after the accident, according to Olivarez' story: he and Dr. Vega have been bleeding the unhappy prince, enlarging the wound twice, and torturing him seemingly on mere guesses. "I believe," says Olivarez, "that all was done well: but as I have said, in wounds in the head there are strange labyrinths." So on the 7th they stand round the bed in despair. Don Garcia de Toledo, the prince's faithful governor, is sitting by him, worn

out with sleepless nights, and trying to supply to the
poor boy that mother's tenderness which he has never
known.   Alva too is there, stern, self-compressed, most
terrible, and yet most beautiful.   He has a God on
earth, and that is Philip his master; and though he
has borne much from Don Carlos already, and will
have to bear more, yet the wretched lad is to him
as a son of God, a second deity, who will by right
divine succeed to the inheritance of the first; and he
watches this lesser deity struggling between life and
death with an intensity of which we, in these less loyal
days, can form no notion.   One would be glad to have
a glimpse of what passed through that mind, so subtle
and so ruthless, so disciplined and so loyal withal: but
Alva was a man who was not given to speak his mind,
but to act it.

One would wish, too, for a glimpse of what was
passing through the mind of another man, who has
been daily in that sick chamber, according to Olivarez'
statement, since the first of the month: but he is one
who has had, for some years past, even more reason
than Alva for not speaking his mind.   What he looked
like we know well, for Titian has painted him from the
life—a tall, bold, well-dressed man, with a noble brain,
square and yet lofty, short curling locks and beard, an
eye which looks as though it feared neither man nor
fiend—and it has had good reason to fear both—and

features which would be exceeding handsome, but for the defiant snub-nose. That is Andreas Vesalius, of Brussels, dreaded and hated by the doctors of the old school—suspect, moreover, it would seem, to inquisitors and theologians, possibly to Alva himself; for he has dared to dissect human bodies; he has insulted the medievalists at Paris, Padua, Bologna, Pisa, Venice, in open theatre; he has turned the heads of all the young surgeons in Italy and France; he has written a great book, with prints in it, designed, some say, by Titian —they were actually done by another Netherlander, John of Calcar, near Cleves—in which he has dared to prove that Galen's anatomy was at fault throughout, and that he had been describing a monkey's inside when he had pretended to be describing a man's; and thus, by impudence and quackery, he has wormed himself—this Netherlander, a heretic at heart, as all Netherlanders are, to God as well as to Galen—into the confidence of the late Emperor Charles V., and gone campaigning with him as one of his physicians, anatomising human bodies even on the battle-field, and defacing the likeness of Deity; and worse than that, the most religious King Philip is deceived by him likewise, and keeps him in Madrid in wealth and honour; and now, in the prince's extreme danger, the king has actually sent for him, and bidden him try his skill—a man who knows nothing save about bones and muscles and the outside of the body, and is unworthy the name of a true physician.

One can conceive the rage of the old Spanish pedants at the Netherlander's appearance, and still more at what followed, if we are to believe Hugo Bloet of Delft, his countryman and contemporary.[*] Vesalius, he says, saw that the surgeons had bound up the wound so tight that an abscess had formed outside the skull, which could not break: he asserted that the only hope lay in opening it; and did so, Philip having given leave, "by two cross-cuts. Then the lad returned to himself, as if awakened from a profound sleep, affirming that he owed his restoration to life to the German doctor."

Dionysius Daza, who was there with the other physicians and surgeons, tells a different story: "The most learned, famous, and rare Baron Vesalius," he says, advised that the skull should be trepanned; but his advice was not followed.

---

[*] I owe this account of Bloet's—which appears to me the only one trustworthy—to the courtesy and erudition of Professor Henry Morley, who finds it quoted from Bloet's 'Acroama,' in the 'Observationum Medicarum Rariorum,' lib. vii., of John Theodore Schenk. Those who wish to know several curious passages of Vesalius' life, which I have not inserted in this article, would do well to consult one by Professor Morley, 'Anatomy in Long Clothes,' in 'Fraser's Magazine' for November, 1853. May I express a hope, which I am sure will be shared by all who have read Professor Morley's biographies of Jerome Carden and of Cornelius Agrippa, that he will find leisure to return to the study of Vesalius' life; and will do for him what he has done for the two just-mentioned writers?

Olivarez' account agrees with that of Daza. They had opened the wounds, he says, down to the skull before Vesalius came. Vesalius insisted that the injury lay inside the skull, and wished to pierce it. Olivarez spends much labour in proving that Vesalius had "no great foundation for his opinion:" but confesses that he never changed that opinion to the last, though all the Spanish doctors were against him. Then on the 6th, he says, the Bachelor Torres came from Madrid, and advised that the skull should be laid bare once more; and on the 7th, there being still doubt whether the skull was not injured, the operation was performed—by whom it is not said—but without any good result, or, according to Olivarez, any discovery, save that Vesalius was wrong, and the skull uninjured.

Whether this second operation of the 7th of May was performed by Vesalius, and whether it was that of which Bloet speaks, is an open question. Olivarez' whole relation is apologetic, written to justify himself and his seven Spanish colleagues, and to prove Vesalius in the wrong. Public opinion, he confesses, had been very fierce against him. The credit of Spanish medicine was at stake: and we are not bound to believe implicitly a paper drawn up under such circumstances for Philip's eye. This, at least, we gather: that Don Carlos was never trepanned, as is commonly said; and this, also, that whichever of the two stories is true, equally puts

Vesalius into direct, and most unpleasant, antagonism
to the Spanish doctors.*

But Don Carlos still lay senseless; and yielding to
popular clamour, the doctors called in the aid of a
certain Moorish doctor, from Valencia, named Priota-
rete, whose unguents, it was reported, had achieved
many miraculous cures. The unguent, however, to the
horror of the doctors, burned the skull till the bone was
as black as the colour of ink; and Olivarez declares he
believes it to have been a preparation of pure caustic.
On the morning of the 9th of May, the Moor and his
unguents were sent away, "and went to Madrid, to
send to heaven Hernando de Vega, while the prince
went back to our method of cure."

Considering what happened on the morning of the
10th of May, we should now presume that the second
opening of the abscess, whether by Vesalius or some one
else, relieved the pressure on the brain; that a critical
period of exhaustion followed, probably prolonged by
the Moor's premature caustic, which stopped the suppu-
ration: but that God's good handiwork, called nature,
triumphed at last; and that therefore it came to pass
that the prince was out of danger within three days of

* Olivarez' 'Relacion' is to be found in the Granvelle State Papers.
For the general account of Don Carlos' illness, and of the miraculous
agencies by which his cure was said to have been effected, the general
reader should consult Miss Frere's 'Biography of Elizabeth of Valois,'
vol. i. pp. 307-19.

the operation. But he was taught, it seems, to attribute his recovery to a very different source from that of a German knife. For on the morning of the 9th, when the Moor was gone, and Don Carlos lay seemingly lifeless, there descended into his chamber a Deus e machinâ, or rather a whole pantheon of greater or lesser deities, who were to effect that which medical skill seemed not to have effected. Philip sent into the prince's chamber several of the precious relics which he usually carried about with him. The miraculous image of the Virgin of Atocha, in embroidering garments for whom, Spanish royalty, male and female, has spent so many an hour ere now, was brought in solemn procession and placed on an altar at the foot of the prince's bed; and in the afternoon there entered, with a procession likewise, a shrine containing the bones of a holy anchorite, one Fray Diego, "whose life and miracles," says Olivarez, "are so notorious;" and the bones of St. Justus and St. Pastor, the tutelar saints of the university of Alcala. Amid solemn litanies the relics of Fray Diego were laid upon the prince's pillow, and the sudarium, or mortuary cloth, which had covered his face, was placed upon the prince's forehead.

Modern science might object that the presence of so many personages, however pious or well intentioned, in a sick chamber on a hot Spanish May day, especially as the bath had been, for some generations past, held in

religious horror throughout Spain, as a sign of Moorish
and Mussulman tendencies, might have somewhat inter-
fered with the chances of the poor boy's recovery.
Nevertheless the event seems to have satisfied Philip's
highest hopes; for that same night (so Don Carlos
afterwards related) the holy monk Diego appeared to
him in a vision, wearing the habit of St. Francis, and
bearing in his hand a cross of reeds tied with a green
band. The prince stated that he first took the appa-
rition to be that of the blessed St. Francis; but not
seeing the stigmata, he exclaimed, "How? Dost thou
not bear the marks of the wounds?" What he replied
Don Carlos did not recollect; save that he consoled him,
and told him that he should not die of that malady.

Philip had returned to Madrid, and shut himself up
in grief in the great Jeronymite monastery. Elizabeth
was praying for her step-son before the miraculous
images of the same city. During the night of the 9th
of May prayers went up for Don Carlos in all the
churches of Toledo, Alcala, and Madrid. Alva stood all
that night at the bed's foot. Don Garcia de Toledo sat
in the arm-chair, where he had now sat night and day
for more than a fortnight. The good preceptor, Hono-
rato Juan, afterwards Bishop of Osma, wrestled in
prayer for the lad the whole night through. His prayer
was answered: probably it had been answered already,
without his being aware of it. Be that as it may, about

dawn Don Carlos' heavy breathing ceased; he fell into a quiet sleep; and when he awoke all perceived at once that he was saved.

He did not recover his sight, seemingly on account of the erysipelas, for a week more. He then opened his eyes upon the miraculous image of Atocha, and vowed that, if he recovered, he would give to the Virgin, at four different shrines in Spain, gold plate of four times his weight; and silver plate of seven times his weight, when he should rise from his couch. So on the 6th of June he rose, and was weighed in a fur coat and a robe of damask, and his weight was three arrobas and one pound—seventy-six pounds in all. On the 14th of June he went to visit his father at the episcopal palace; then to all the churches and shrines in Alcala, and of course to that of Fray Diego, whose body it is said he contemplated for some time with edifying devotion. The next year saw Fray Diego canonised as a saint, at the intercession of Philip and his son; and thus Don Carlos reentered the world, to be a terror and a torment to all around him, and to die—not by Philip's cruelty, as his enemies reported too hastily indeed, yet excusably, for they knew him to be capable of any wickedness—but simply of constitutional insanity.

And now let us go back to the history of "that most learned, famous, and rare Baron Vesalius," who had stood by and seen all these things done; and try if we cannot, after we have learned the history of his early life, guess at some of his probable meditations on this celebrated clinical case; and guess also how those meditations may have affected seriously the events of his after life.

Vesalius (as I said) was a Netherlander, born at Brussels in 1513 or 1514. His father and grandfather had been medical men of the highest standing in a profession which then, as now, was commonly hereditary. His real name was Wittag, an ancient family of Wesel, on the Rhine, from which town either he or his father adopted the name of Vesalius, according to the classicising fashion of those days. Young Vesalius was sent to college at Louvain, where he learned rapidly. At sixteen or seventeen he knew not only Latin, but Greek enough to correct the proofs of Galen, and Arabic enough to become acquainted with the works of the Mussulman physicians. He was a physicist, too, and a mathematician, according to the knowledge of those times; but his passion—the study to which he was destined to devote his life—was anatomy.

Little or nothing (it must be understood) had been done in anatomy since the days of Galen of Pergamos, in the second century after Christ, and very little even by him. Dissection was all but forbidden among the ancients. The Egyptians, Herodotus tells us, used to pursue with stones and curses the embalmers as soon as they had performed their unpleasant office; and though Herophilus and Erasistratus are said to have dissected many subjects under the protection of Ptolemy Soter in Alexandria itself: yet the public feeling of the Greeks as well as of the Romans continued the same as that of the ancient Egyptians; and Galen was fain—as Vesalius proved—to supplement his ignorance of the human frame by describing that of an ape. Dissection was equally forbidden among the Mussulmans; and the great Arabic physicians could do no more than comment on Galen. The same prejudice extended through the middle age. Medical men were all clerks, clerici, and as such forbidden to shed blood. The only dissection, as far as I am aware, made during the middle age was one by Mundinus in 1306; and his subsequent commentaries on Galen—for he dare allow his own eyes to see no more than Galen had seen before him—constituted the best anatomical manual in Europe till the middle of the fifteenth century.

Then, in Italy at least, the classic Renaissance gave fresh life to anatomy as to all other sciences. Especially did the improvements in painting and sculpture stir men up to a closer study of the human frame. Leonardo da Vinci wrote a treatise on muscular anatomy: the artist and the sculptor often worked together, and realised that sketch of Michael Angelo's in which he himself is assisting Fallopius, Vesalius' famous

pupil, to dissect. Vesalius soon found that his thirst
for facts could not be slaked by the theories of the
middle age ; so in 1530 he went off to Montpellier,
where Francis I. had just founded a medical school,
and where the ancient laws of the city allowed the
faculty each year the body of a criminal. From thence,
after becoming the fellow-pupil and the friend of
Rondelet, and probably also of Rabelais and those other
luminaries of Montpellier, of whom I spoke in my essay
on Rondelet, he returned to Paris to study under old
Sylvius, whose real name was Jacques Dubois, *alias*
Jock o' the Wood ; and to learn less—as he complains
himself—in an anatomical theatre than a butcher might
learn in his shop.

Were it not that the whole question of dissection
is one over which it is right to draw a reverent veil, as
a thing painful, however necessary and however innocent, it would be easy to raise ghastly laughter in
many a reader by the stories which Vesalius himself
tells of his struggles to learn anatomy.—How old
Sylvius tried to demonstrate the human frame from
a bit of a dog, fumbling in vain for muscles which he
could not find, or which ought to have been there,
according to Galen, and were not; while young
Vesalius, as soon as the old pedant's back was turned,
took his place, and, to the delight of the students,
found for him—provided it were there—what he could

not find himself;—how he went body-snatching and gibbet-robbing, often at the danger of his life, as when he and his friend were nearly torn to pieces by the cannibal dogs who haunted the Butte de Montfaucon, or place of public execution;—how he acquired, by a long and dangerous process, the only perfect skeleton then in the world, and the hideous story of the robber to whom it had belonged—all these horrors those who list may read for themselves elsewhere. I hasten past them with this remark—that to have gone through the toils, dangers, and disgusts which Vesalius faced, argued in a superstitious and cruel age like his, no common physical and moral courage, and a deep conscience that he was doing right, and must do it at all risks in the face of a generation which, peculiarly reckless of human life and human agony, allowed that frame which it called the image of God to be tortured, maimed, desecrated in every way while alive; and yet—straining at the gnat after having swallowed the camel—forbade it to be examined when dead, though for the purpose of alleviating the miseries of mankind.

The breaking out of war between Francis I. and Charles V. drove Vesalius back to his native country and Louvain; and in 1535 we hear of him as a surgeon in Charles V.'s army. He saw, most probably, the Emperor's invasion of Provence, and the

disastrous retreat from before Montmorency's forti-
fied camp at Avignon, through a country in which
that crafty general had destroyed every article of
human food, except the half-ripe grapes. He saw,
perhaps, the Spanish soldiers, poisoned alike by the
sour fruit and by the blazing sun, falling in hundreds
along the white roads which led back into Savoy,
murdered by the peasantry whose homesteads had been
destroyed, stifled by the weight of their own armour, or
desperately putting themselves, with their own hands,
out of a world which had become intolerable. Half
the army perished. Two thousand corpses lay festering
between Aix and Fréjus alone. If young Vesalius
needed "subjects," the ambition and the crime of man
found enough for him in those blazing September days.

He went to Italy, probably with the remnants of
the army. Where could he have rather wished to
find himself? He was at last in the country where
the human mind seemed to be growing young once
more; the country of revived arts, revived sciences,
learning, languages; and—though, alas, only for a
while—of revived free thought, such as Europe had
not seen since the palmy days of Greece. Here at
least he would be appreciated; here at least he would
be allowed to think and speak: and he was appreciated.
The Italian cities, who were then, like the Athenians of
old, " spending their time in nothing else save to hear

or to tell something new," welcomed the brave young Fleming and his novelties. Within two years he was professor of anatomy at Padua, then the first school in the world; then at Bologna and at Pisa at the same time; last of all at Venice, where Titian painted that portrait of him which remains unto this day.

These years were for him a continual triumph; everywhere, as he demonstrated on the human body, students crowded his theatre, or hung round him as he walked the streets; professors left their own chairs—their scholars having deserted them already —to go and listen humbly or enviously to the man who could give them what all brave souls throughout half Europe were craving for, and craving in vain: facts. And so, year after year, was realised that scene which stands engraved in the frontispiece of his great book—where, in the little quaint Cinquecento theatre, saucy scholars, reverend doctors, gay gentlemen, and even cowled monks, are crowding the floor, peeping over each other's shoulders, hanging on the balustrades; while in the centre, over his " subject "— which one of those same cowled monks knew but too well —stands young Vesalius, upright, proud, almost defiant, as one who knows himself safe in the impregnable citadel of fact; and in his hand the little blade of steel, destined—because wielded in obedience to the

2 D

laws of nature, which are the laws of God—to work more benefit for the human race than all the swords which were drawn in those days, or perhaps in any other, at the bidding of most Catholic Emperors and most Christian Kings.

Those were indeed days of triumph for Vesalius; of triumph deserved, because earned by patient and accurate toil in a good cause: but Vesalius, being but a mortal man, may have contracted in those same days a temper of imperiousness and self-conceit, such as he showed afterwards when his pupil Fallopius dared to add fresh discoveries to those of his master. And yet, in spite of all Vesalius knew, how little he knew! How humbling to his pride it would have been had he known then—perhaps he does know now—that he had actually again and again walked, as it were, round and round the true theory of the circulation of the blood, and yet never seen it; that that discovery which, once made, is intelligible, as far as any phenomenon is intelligible, to the merest peasant, was reserved for another century, and for one of those Englishmen on whom Vesalius would have looked as semi-barbarians.

To make a long story short: three years after the publication of his famous book, 'De Corporis Humani Fabrica,' he left Venice to cure Charles V., at Regensburg, and became one of the great Emperor's physicians.

This was the crisis of Vesalius' life. The medicine with which he had worked the cure was China— Sarsaparilla, as we call it now—brought home from the then newly-discovered banks of the Paraguay and Uruguay, where its beds of tangled vine, they say, tinge the clear waters a dark brown like that of peat, and convert whole streams into a healthful and pleasant tonic. On the virtues of this China (then supposed to be a root) Vesalius wrote a famous little book, into which he contrived to interweave his opinions on things in general, as good Bishop Berkeley did afterwards into his essay on the virtues of tar-water. Into this book, however, Vesalius introduced—as Bishop Berkeley did not—much, and perhaps too much, about himself; and much, though perhaps not too much, about poor old Galen, and his substitution of an ape's inside for that of a human being. The storm which had been long gathering burst upon him. The old school, trembling for their time-honoured reign, bespattered, with all that pedantry, ignorance, and envy could suggest, the man who dared not only to revolutionise surgery, but to interfere with the privileged mysteries of medicine; and, over and above, to become a favourite at the court of the greatest of monarchs. While such as Eustachius, himself an able discoverer, could join in the cry, it is no wonder if a lower soul, like that of Sylvius, led it open-mouthed. He was a mean, covetous, bad man, as George Buchanan well knew; and, according to his nature, he wrote a furious book, 'Ad Vesani calumnias depulsandas.' The punning change of Vesalius into Vesanus (madman) was but a fair and gentle stroke for a polemic, in days in which those who could not kill their enemies with steel or powder, held themselves justified in doing so, if possible, by vituperation, calumny, and every engine of moral torture. But a far more terrible weapon, and one which made Vesalius rage, and it may be for once in his life tremble, was the charge of impiety and heresy. The Inquisition was a very ugly place. It was very easy to get into it, especially for a Netherlander: but not so easy to get out. Indeed Vesalius must have trembled, when he saw his master, Charles V., himself take fright, and actually call on the theologians of Salamanca to decide whether it was lawful to dissect a human body. The monks, to their honour, used their common sense, and answered Yes. The deed was so plainly useful, that it must be lawful likewise. But Vesalius did not feel that he had triumphed. He dreaded, possibly, lest the storm should only have blown over for a time. He fell, possibly, into hasty disgust at the folly of mankind, and despair of arousing them to use their common sense, and acknowledge their true interest and their true benefactors. At all events, he threw into the fire—so it is said—all his unpublished manuscripts, the records of long years of observation, and renounced science thenceforth.

We hear of him after this at Brussels, and at Basle likewise—in which latter city, in the company of physicians, naturalists, and Grecians, he must have breathed awhile a freer air. But he seems to have returned thence to his old master Charles V., and to have finally settled at Madrid as a court surgeon to Philip II., who sent him, but too late, to extract the lance splinters from the eye of the dying Henry II.

He was now married to a lady of rank from Brussels, Anne van Hamme by name; and their daughter married in time Philip II.'s grand falconer, who was doubtless a personage of no small social rank. He was well off in worldly things; somewhat fond, it is said, of good living and of luxury; inclined, it may be, to say, "Let us eat and drink, for to-morrow we die," and to sink more and more into the mere worldling, unless some shock awoke him from his lethargy.

And the awakening shock did come. After eight years of court life, he resolved early in the year 1564 to go on pilgrimage to Jerusalem.

The reasons for so strange a determination are wrapped in mystery and contradiction. The common story was that he had opened a corpse to ascertain

2 D 3

the cause of death, and that, to the horror of the
bystanders, the heart was still seen to beat; that his
enemies accused him to the Inquisition, and that he
was condemned to death, a sentence which was com-
muted to that of going on pilgrimage. But here,
at the very outset, accounts differ. One says that
the victim was a nobleman, name not given; another
that it was a lady's maid, name not given. It is most
improbable, if not impossible, that Vesalius, of all men,
should have mistaken a living body for a dead one;
while it is most probable, on the other hand, that his
medical enemies would gladly raise such a calumny
against him, when he was no longer in Spain to contradict it. Meanwhile Llorente, the historian of the
Inquisition, makes no mention of Vesalius having been
brought before its tribunal, while he does mention
Vesalius' residence at Madrid. Another story is, that
he went abroad to escape the bad temper of his wife;
another that he wanted to enrich himself. Another
story—and that not an unlikely one—is, that he was
jealous of the rising reputation of his pupil Fallopius,
then professor of anatomy at Venice. This distinguished
surgeon, as I said before, had written a book, in which
he had added to Vesalius' discoveries, and corrected
certain errors of his. Vesalius had answered him
hastily and angrily, quoting his anatomy from memory;
for, as he himself complained, he could not in Spain

obtain a subject for dissection; not even, he said, a single skull. He had sent his book to Venice to be published, and had heard, seemingly, nothing of it. He may have felt that he was falling behind in the race of science, and that it was impossible for him to carry on his studies in Madrid; and so, angry with his own laziness and luxury, he may have felt the old sacred fire flash up in him, and have determined to go to Italy and become a student and a worker once more.

The very day that he set out, Clusius of Arras, then probably the best botanist in the world, arrived at Madrid; and, asking the reason of Vesalius' departure, was told by their fellow-countryman, Charles de Tisnacq, procurator for the affairs of the Netherlands, that Vesalius had gone of his own free will, and with all facilities which Philip could grant him, in performance of a vow which he had made during a dangerous illness. Here, at least, we have a drop of information, which seems taken from the stream sufficiently near to the fountain-head: but it must be recollected that De Tisnacq lived in dangerous times, and may have found it necessary to walk warily in them; that through him had been sent, only the year before, that famous letter from William of Orange, Horn, and Egmont, the fate whereof may be read in Mr. Motley's fourth chapter; that the crisis of the Netherlands which sprung out of that letter was coming fast; and that, as De Tisnacq was on friendly terms with Egmont, he may have felt his head at times somewhat loose on his shoulders; especially if he had heard Alva say, as he wrote, " that every time he saw the despatches of those three señors, they moved his choler so, that if he did not take much care to temper it, he would seem a frenzied man." In such times, De Tisnacq may have thought good to return a diplomatic answer to a fellow-countryman concerning a third fellow-countryman, especially when that countryman, as a former pupil of Melancthon at Wittemberg, might himself be under suspicion of heresy, and therefore of possible treason.

Be this as it may, one cannot but suspect some strain of truth in the story about the Inquisition; perhaps in that, also, of his wife's unkindness; for, whether or not Vesalius operated on Don Calos, he had seen with his own eyes that miraculous Virgin of Atocha at the bed's foot of the prince. He had heard his recovery attri buted, not to the operation, but to the intercession of Fray, now Saint, Diego; * and he must have had his thoughts thereon, and may, in an unguarded moment, have spoken them.

---

* In justice to poor Doctor Olivarez, it must be said, that while he allows all force to the intercession of the Virgin and of Fray Diego, and of "many just persons," he cannot allow that there was any "miracle properly so called," because the prince was cured according to "natural order," and by "experimented remedies" of the physicians.

For he was, be it always remembered, a Netherlander. The crisis of his country was just at hand.
Rebellion was inevitable, and, with rebellion, horrors
unutterable; and, meanwhile, Don Carlos had set his
mad brain on having the command of the Netherlands.
In his rage at not having it, as all the world knows,
he nearly killed Alva with his own hands, some two
years after. If it be true that Don Carlos felt a
debt of gratitude to Vesalius, he may (after his wont)
have poured out to him some wild confidence about
the Netherlands, to have even heard which would be
a crime in Philip's eyes. And if this be but a fancy,
still Vesalius was, as I just said, a Netherlander, and
one of a brain and a spirit to which Philip's doings, and
the air of the Spanish court, must have been growing
even more and more intolerable. Hundreds of his
country folk, perhaps men and women whom he had
known, were being racked, burnt alive, buried alive, at
the bidding of a jocular ruffian, Peter Titelmann, the
chief inquisitor. The "day of the *mau-brulez*," and
the wholesale massacre which followed it, had happened but two years before; and, by all the signs of
the times, these murders and miseries were certain to
increase. And why were all these poor wretches suffering the extremity of horror, but because they would
not believe in miraculous images, and bones of dead
friars, and the rest of that science of unreason and

unfact, against which Vesalius had been fighting all his life, consciously or not, by using reason and observing fact? What wonder if, in some burst of noble indignation and just contempt, he forgot a moment that he had sold his soul, and his love of science likewise, to be a luxurious, yet uneasy, hanger-on at the tyrant's court; and spoke unadvisedly some word worthy of a German man?

As to the story of his unhappy quarrels with his wife, there may be a grain of truth in it likewise. Vesalius' religion must have sat very lightly on him. The man who had robbed churchyards and gibbets from his youth was not likely to be much afraid of apparitions and demons. He had handled too many human bones to care much for those of saints. He was probably, like his friends of Basle, Montpellier, and Paris, somewhat of a heretic at heart, probably somewhat of a pagan. His lady, Anne van Hamme, was probably a strict Catholic, as her father, being a councillor and master of the exchequer at Brussels, was bound to be; and freethinking in the husband, crossed by superstition in the wife, may have caused in them that wretched vie à part, that want of any true communion of soul, too common to this day in Catholic countries.

Be these things as they may—and the exact truth of them will now be never known—Vesalius set out to Jerusalem in the spring of 1564. On his way he

visited his old friends at Venice to see about his book
against Fallopius. The Venetian republic received the
great philosopher with open arms. Fallopius was just
dead; and the senate offered their guest the vacant
chair of anatomy. He accepted it: but went on to the
East.

He never occupied that chair; wrecked upon the
Isle of Zante, as he was sailing back from Palestine, he
died miserably of fever and want, as thousands of pilgrims returning from the Holy Land had died before
him. A goldsmith recognised him; buried him in a
chapel of the Virgin; and put up over him a simple
stone, which remained till late years; and may remain,
for aught I know, even now.

So perished, in the prime of life, "a martyr to his
love of science," to quote the words of M. Burggraeve
of Ghent, his able biographer and commentator, "the
prodigious man, who created a science at an epoch
when everything was still an obstacle to his progress;
a man whose whole life was a long struggle of knowledge against ignorance, of truth against lies."

Plaudite: Exeat: with Rondelet and Buchanan. And
whensoever this poor foolish world needs three such
men, may God of his great mercy send them.

LONDON:
PRINTED BY WILLIAM CLOWES AND SONS, LIMITED,
STAMFORD STREET AND CHARING CROSS.

www.ingramcontent.com/pod-product-compliance
Lightning Source LLC
Chambersburg PA
CBHW032312280326
41932CB00009B/784